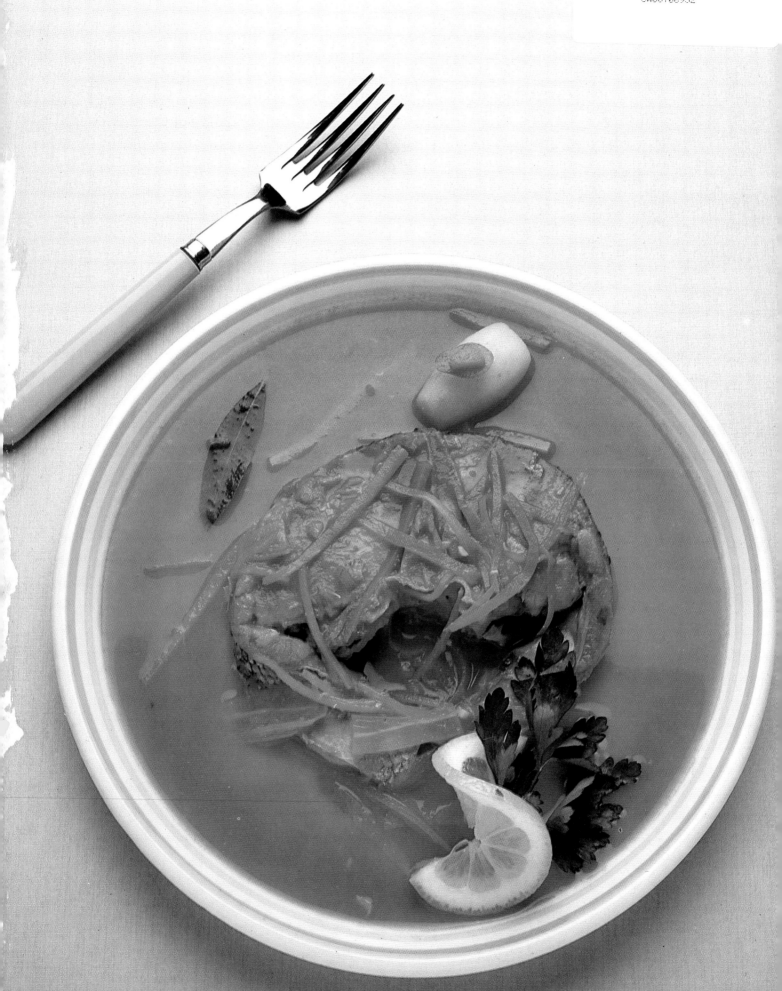

This edition first published in 1993 by
Sunburst Books, Deacon House, 65 Old Church Street,
London, SW3 5BS

Copyright © Editorial LIBSA, Narciso Serra, 25 – Tel 433 54 07 –
28007 MADRID
4.ª EDICION 1991
Copyright English language text © 1993 Sunburst Books

ISBN 1 85778 005 1

Printed and bound in China

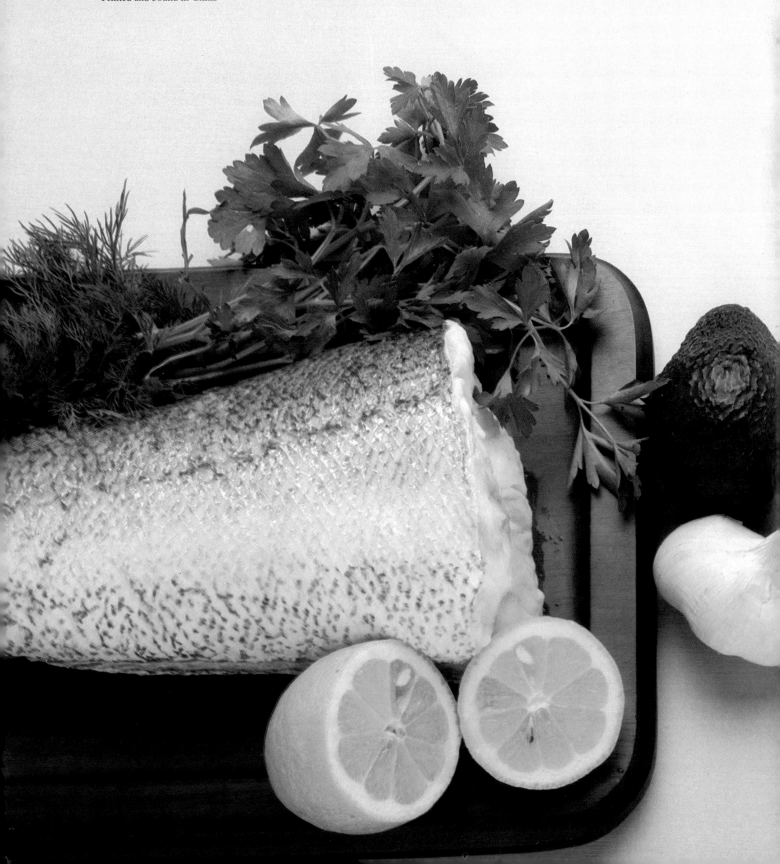

SLIMMER'S COOKBOOK

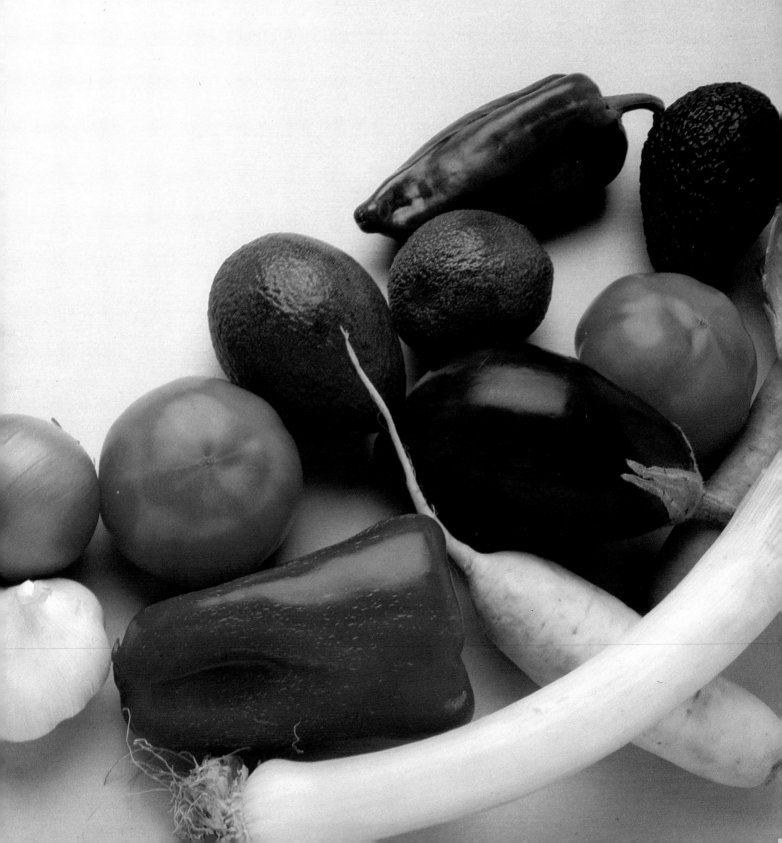

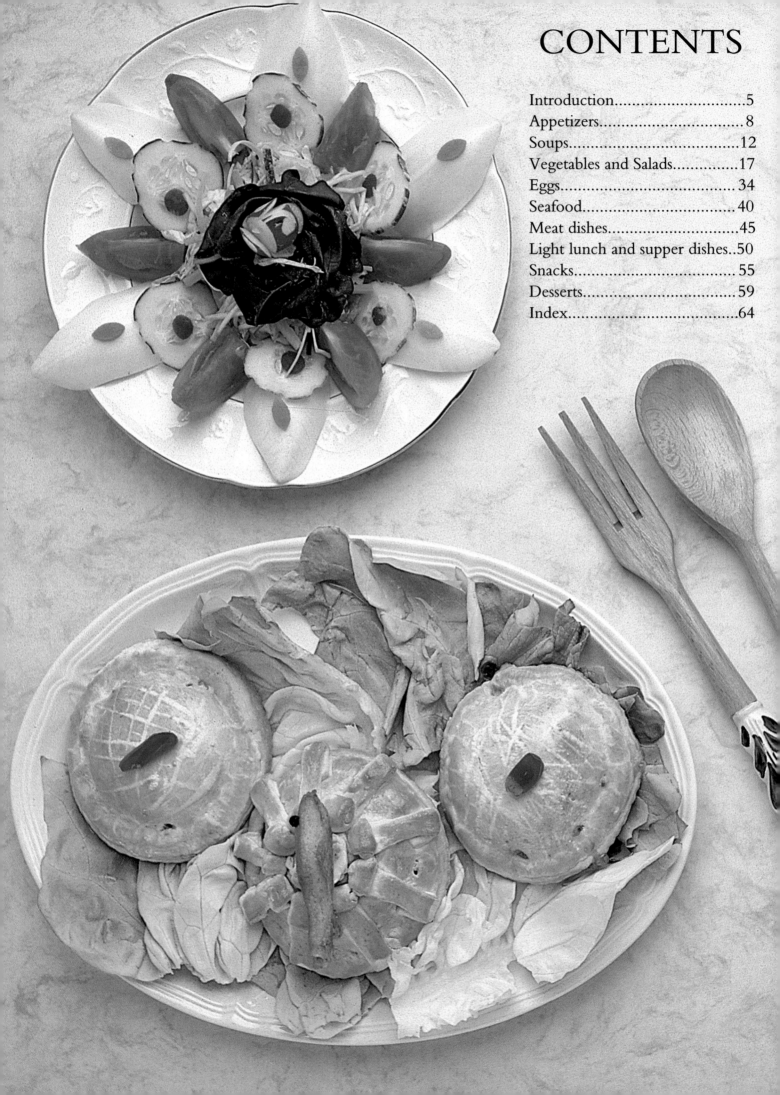

CONTENTS

INTRODUCTION

A diet designed for weight loss conjures up images of unappetizing vegetable dishes or endless grilled chicken. However, cookery is the art of transforming eating for survival into eating for pleasure, and it can also transform a low-calorie diet into a pleasurable experience.

Foods contain an energy value, which is produced when the human body "burns" its nutritional components and it is measured in calories. There are some food components which do not contain any calorific value - for example, vitamins, minerals, vegetable fibre and water. However, although they are not energy providers, they fulfil important roles in the body.

The elements which have a calorific value - or energy - within food components are as follows:

Protein	1g = 4 calories
Carbohydrates	1g = 4 calories
Fat	1g = 9 calories

Clearly, fat is the source of most energy. Humans require a certain level of energy to carry out daily activities, as well as for growth and reproduction functions.
This requirement depends on body area, age and sex.

In general energy requirements are as follows:

Young Men	3,000 calories per day
Adult Men	2,700 calories per day
Young Women	2,100 calories per day
Adult Women	2,000 calories per day

To lose weight, an energy imbalance must be created - that is, the calories consumed must be less than those needed, so that consumption of calorie reserves results in progressive weight loss, but without endangering health. This is very important, as weight loss should not lead to weakness or a risk of illness. So the reduced diet must be balanced and should contain balanced proportions of proteins, fats and carbohydrates. Food contains these three fundamental components in different proportions. Some contain a large quantity of protein, such as meat, fish, eggs and dairy products; some, such as butter and oil, are a source of fat; while others have a high proportion of carbohydrates - for example, potatoes, flour and cereals.

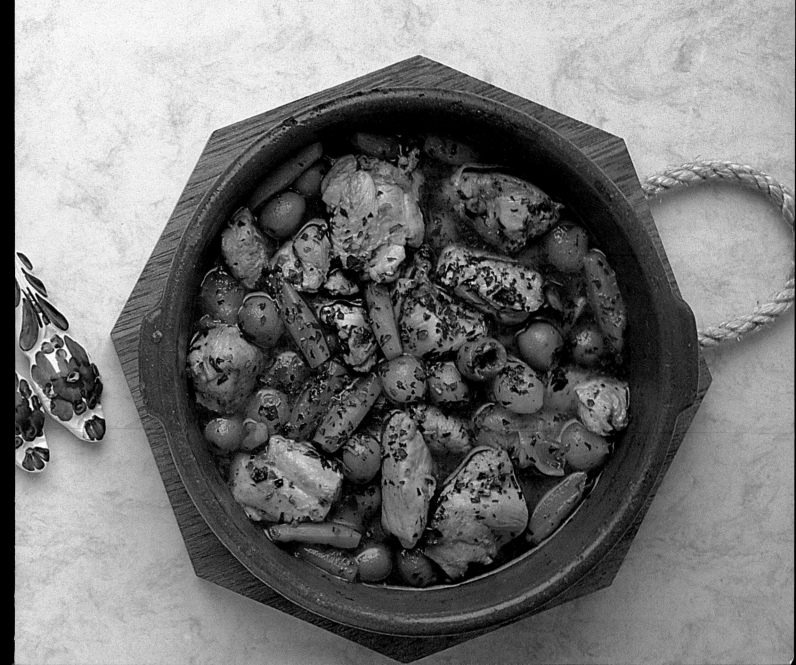

If foods are categorised according to their contents they can be divided into seven groups:

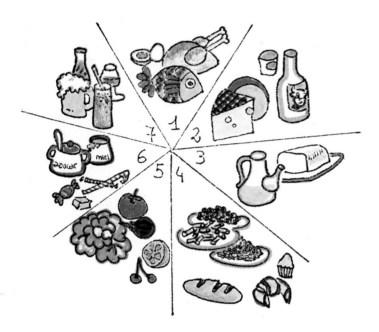

A balanced diet must provide food from all these groups. A deficiency of foodstuffs from one of the groups would result in an unbalanced and unhealthy diet.

Recipes are measured per person, working out the weight of the raw ingredients. The breakdown of proteins, fats and carbohydrates is also provided alongside each recipe. By adding up what each recipe or food eaten during the day provides in terms of food components, you can determine whether or not you have a balanced diet.

The following percentages are recommended:

Protein : 10-20% of the total calorific value
Carbohydrate : 50-60% of the total calorific value
Fat : 20-30% of the total calorific value

To work out this percentage in grammes, assume that, in a daily intake of 1000 calories, there should be:

50-60g protein
125-150g carbohydrate
20-30g fat

All the recipes have been devised using natural products. None of the recipes include low-calorie products, skimmed milk or artificial sweeteners, because cooking to lose weight should be healthy and varied and should not deviate too far from normal nutritional habits. It is far more effective to address excesses and to moderate food intake. The following comments should provide some useful pointers:

1. A diet to lose weight should only be a temporary necessity, so it is worth making changes to our ordinary diet to avoid potentially unhealthy and harmful excesses.
2. We have seen that the nutritional element with the highest

calorific value is fat, so we should look for ways of reducing it, bearing in mind that:

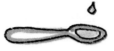

1 tablespoon oil (10g) = 90 cal.

which is equivalent to:

3 slices of bread 1cm thick = 90 cal.

150g apple = 90 cal.

1 egg = 80 cal.

1 chocolate sweet = 90 cal

So it is advisable to:

• Reduce the oil in dressings for vegetables and salads by using seasonings which do not contain many calories, such as vinegar, lemon juice, spices and aromatic herbs
• Remove the fat from soups, broths and stews: if you leave the soup or stew to cool, it is easy to skim off the fat which rises to the surface. Therefore extra time must be allowed when cooking
• Remove fat from meat and avoid those meats which have a high fat content such as pork and pork products
• Avoid sweets and chocolate with a high fat content (They also have a high sugar content)
• Eat fish! Fat intake is reduced if meat is replaced by fish:

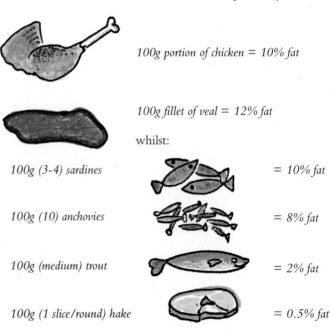

100g portion of chicken = 10% fat

100g fillet of veal = 12% fat

whilst:

100g (3-4) sardines   *= 10% fat*

100g (10) anchovies   *= 8% fat*

100g (medium) trout   *= 2% fat*

100g (1 slice/round) hake   *= 0.5% fat*

although it is true that fish often seems less filling than meat. **NB.** The calorific value of margarine is almost the same as butter, as with all the seed based oils, such as olive, sunflower, corn.

3. Water intake should not be reduced, although if liquid retention is a problem, it is advisable to drink between meals, rather than at mealtimes themselves.

4. Toast has a similar calorific value to ordinary bread - toasting does not alter the nutritional value .

5. Take care with canapés and snacks: they can contain a high amount of energy.

For example:

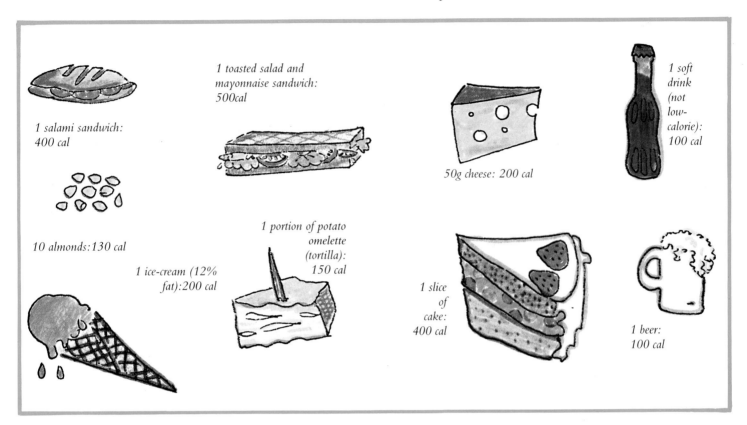

1 salami sandwich: 400 cal

1 toasted salad and mayonnaise sandwich: 500cal

10 almonds:130 cal

1 ice-cream (12% fat):200 cal

1 portion of potato omelette (tortilla): 150 cal

50g cheese: 200 cal

1 slice of cake: 400 cal

1 soft drink (not low-calorie): 100 cal

1 beer: 100 cal

But ....

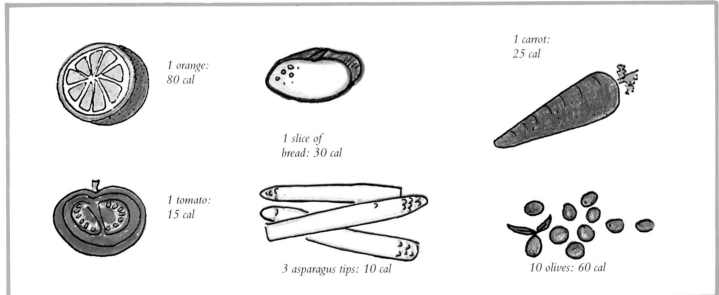

1 orange: 80 cal

1 slice of bread: 30 cal

1 carrot: 25 cal

1 tomato: 15 cal

3 asparagus tips: 10 cal

10 olives: 60 cal

6. It is not advisable to "skip" any of the three standard meals - breakfast, lunch, dinner - an occasional excess will be corrected by moderation, not by an imbalanced, sporadic diet.

7. It is recommended to eat slowly, as one only feels replete 10-20 minutes after eating. It also promotes more effective digestion

The recipes provided here have different calorific values and some cannot be used in very strict diets - but the majority will be a valuable resource when planning healthy and appetizing menus for weight loss.

APPETIZERS

The hour of aperitifs or, more precisely, of pre-dinner drinks and appetizers, presents a moment of temptation which can knock a diet off course. To overcome this potential temptation, some low calorie snacks are provided below. Although, obviously, if 1 canapé has, for example, 40 calories, 4 will have 160 calories.... and you will have to add this to the total for the rest of the food eaten during the day. However, because they are consumed in such small quantities, appetizers will not have any considerable affect on the nutritional elements - they are more of a treat than a source of nutrition.

VARIOUS CANAPÉS

1 piece of bread (fresh or toasted), with
Tomato
Anchovy

Cover the bread with a small slice of tomato and garnish with the washed anchovy.
Cal. 40

Tomato
Boiled egg

Cover the bread with a slice of tomato and then a slice of boiled egg.
Cal. 40

Ham
Cheese spread

Spread the cheese on the bread and cover with a slice of ham.
Cal. 45

Smoked Salmon
Lemon

Place the smoked salmon, without oil, on the bread and garnish with a small piece of lemon.
Cal. 40

Soft cheese
Gherkin slices

Spread the cheese on the bread and garnish with the gherkin slices.
Cal. 40

Carrots
Gherkin slices

Grate the carrots and chop the gherkin slices finely. Mix and place on the bread. Cheese can also be added.
Cal. 35

Asparagus
Anchovy

Wash the anchovy and spread it onto the bread, place the asparagus tip on top.
Cal. 40

Cottage Cheese
Cinnamon
Pineapple

Cover the bread with cottage cheese, sprinkle with cinnamon and decorate with pineapple.
Cal. 45

Soft Cheese
Anchovy

Spread the cheese on the bread and garnish with fine strips of anchovy (washed and drained).
Cal. 45

VARIOUS BITE-SIZED SNACKS

1 small slice of tomato
1 anchovy

Wash the anchovy and roll it around the tomato slice.
Cal. 20

1 slice tomato
1 cube cheese

Thread both onto a cocktail stick.
Cal. 15

Slice of beetroot in vinegar
Gherkin slice

Thread both onto a cocktail stick.
Cal. 10

Spring onion
Gherkin slice

Thread both onto a cocktail stick.
Cal. 10

Celery
Carrot

Wash and peel the carrot and celery. Cut a long slice of carrot and a smaller one of celery and thread them onto a cocktail stick.
Cal. 10

1 slice York Ham
3 slices gherkin
Slice sweet pepper

Thread the three ingredients onto a cocktail stick.
Cal. 15

GHERKIN WITH HAM

1 large gherkin
1 slice York ham
1 slice sweet pepper

Cut the gherkin into slices and alternate it with the York ham and pepper, fixing with a cocktail stick.
Cal. 40

Various Canapés

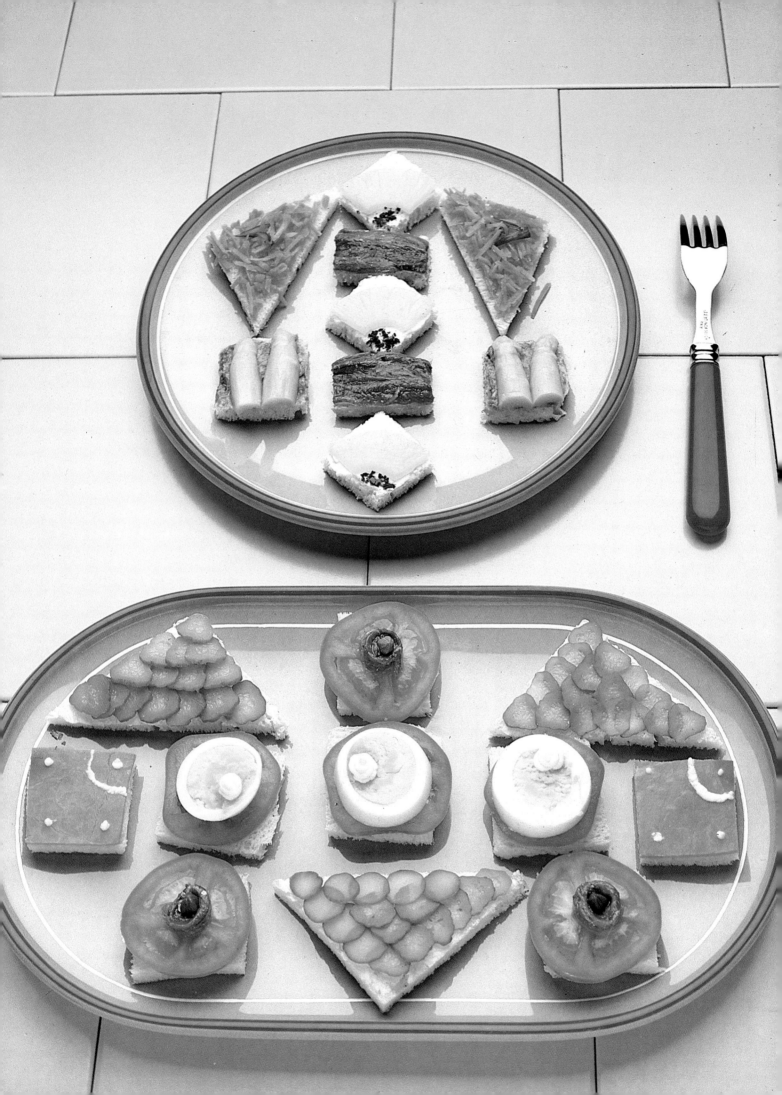

ANCHOVY WITH GHERKIN

1 large gherkin in vinegar
1 anchovy

Wash the anchovy if it is in oil. Cut the gherkin in half lengthways and stuff with the anchovy.

This can also be done with a small piece of roast or grilled chicken.
Cal. 30

PRUNES WITH CHEESE

1 prune
spoonful soft cheese

Take the stone out of the prune and stuff with the soft cheese or with York ham.
Cal. 45

ANCHOVIES IN VINEGAR

¹/₂ kg / 1 lb anchovies
¹/₄ litre / ¹/₂ pint vinegar
Parsley
Salt

Clean the anchovies, taking out the back bone and separating them into 2 fillets. Wash well and leave overnight in vinegar. The following day, drain and put them into fresh vinegar with salt and chopped parsley.

If they are kept for more than 2 days, the vinegar should be removed and they must be covered in oil, but wash off the oil before eating, due to its high calorific content.
1 anchovy: Cal. 15

HAM AND PINEAPPLE CHUNKS

1 chunk pineapple
1 thin slice York ham

Wrap the ham around the pineapple chunk and thread onto a cocktail stick. Serve cold or warm.
Cal. 30

HAM AND BAGUETTES

1 slice French bread
1 thin slice York ham

Wrap the York ham around the slice of bread, leaving the 2 ends of the slice of bread showing edges.
Cal. 35

Bite–sized snacks

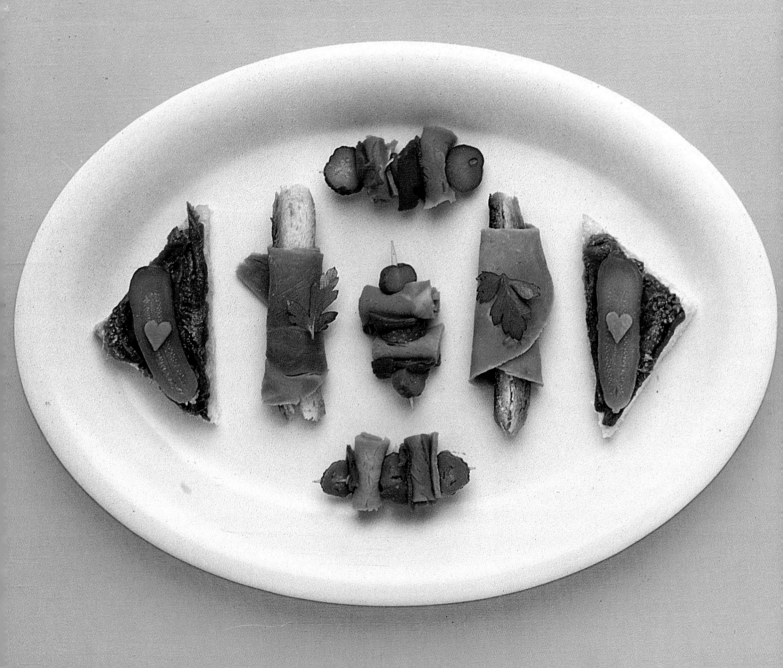

CHEESE AND ORANGE SLICE

1 slice orange
1 cube cheese

Peel the orange and slice, removing all the pith. Anchor orange slice on a cube of cheese using a cocktail stick.
Cal. 15

APPLE AND ANCHOVY SLICE

1 slice apple
1 lemon
1 anchovy

Rub the apple slice with the lemon so it does not turn brown. Wash the anchovy to remove the oil. Wrap the anchovy around the apple and fix in place with the cocktail stick.
Cal. 40

Canapés

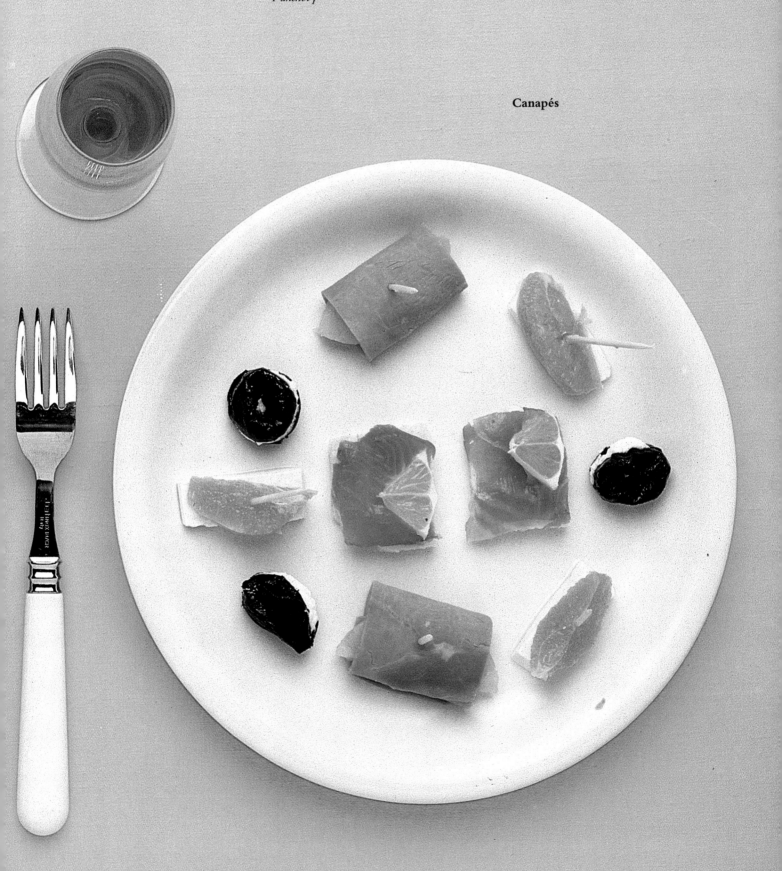

SOUPS

Soups made by the traditional method of simmering a combination of ingredients, and even some commercially produced soups can be quite low in calories, provided they contain no fat. In fact, both commercially produced and traditional (home-made) soups usually do contain fat, - but this can be addressed if they are left to cool and the fat which rises to the surface is skimmed off. This fat comes from the meat or meat stock used to make the soup. The soups in this chapter do not contain much butter, cream or oil. The recipe for gazpacho; can be substituted by other recipes, provided they only use a limited quantity of oil and bread.

Left, top: Gazpacho
Left, bottom: Vichyssoise
Opposite, top: Fish Soup(recipe on page 14)
Opposite, bottom: Italian Soup with Cheese

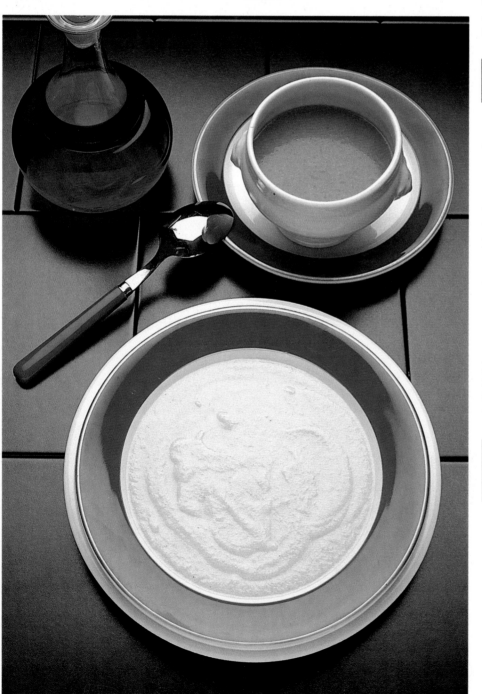

ITALIAN SOUP WITH CHEESE

2 litres stock (home-made or cube)
50g celery
200g carrots
300g cabbage, sliced
100g potato, cubed
100g grated cheese (Parmesan, Gruyère)

Wash the celery and cut it into strips. Clean the carrots and grate finely. Cook all the vegetables in the stock for 30 minutes. Add the grated cheese just before serving, and serve piping hot.

	Cal.	Pro.	Fat	Carbo.
Per Serving	154	4.1	9	14

GAZPACHO

1 kg ripe tomatoes
100g cucumber
50g pepper
20g bread
3 tablespoons oil
1 tablespoon vinegar
1 litre cold water
salt

To garnish:
100g tomato
100g green pepper

Blend all the ingredients in an electric mixer or food processor and then sieve. Serve cold, garnished with finely chopped tomatoes and green pepper.

	Cal.	Pro.	Fat	Carbo.
Per Serving	144	3.2	8.4	13.9
Per Garnish	15	0.07	0.15	3

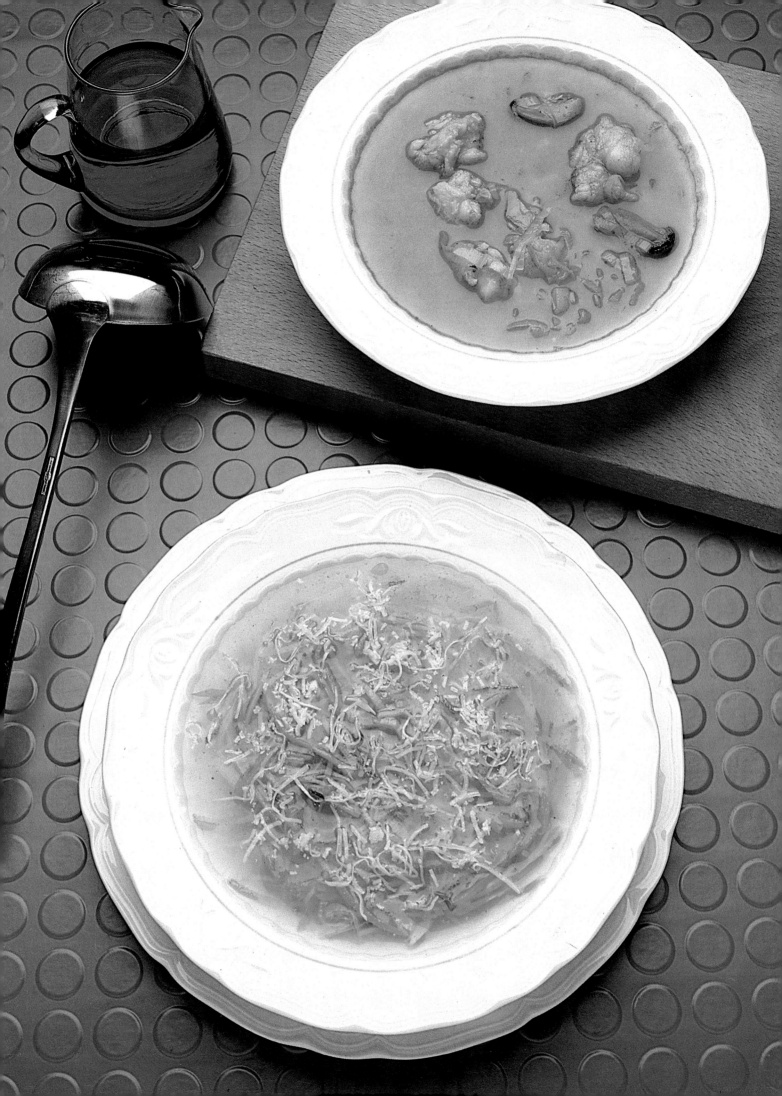

FISH SOUP

¹/₂ kg fish (hake, eel)
¹/₂ kg mussels
200g leeks
2 carrots, sliced
1 onion, quartered
2 tablespoons oil
2 cloves garlic, chopped
sprig parsley
2 bay leaves
thyme
juice of ¹/₂ lemon

Make a fish stock by putting the fish bones into 2 litres of water and adding the onion, carrot, parsley, bay leaves. Cook for 30 minutes and then strain. Open the mussels by putting them in a pan with a little water, salt and lemon juice and heating gently. Take out the mussels and keep the drained stock.

Fry the garlic in the oil until golden and then add the finely chopped leek and sauté until soft. Add the stock from the fish and mussels. After cooking for a few minutes add the chopped fish, and bring to the boil. Simmer for a few more minutes, then remove from the heat, add the mussels and serve.

	Cal.	Pro.	Fat	Carbo.
Per Serving	177	24.7	5.8	6.6

VICHYSSOISE

1 litre stock (home-made or cube)
400g leeks, cleaned and chopped
200g potatoes, cubed
100ml single cream
salt

Cook the leek and potatoes with the stock for 20 minutes. Blend using a sieve or food processor. Heat through, add salt to taste and add the single cream.

This soup can be served hot or cold, sprinkled with chopped parsley.

	Cal.	Pro.	Fat	Carbo.
Per Serving	135	3.3	6.3	14.3

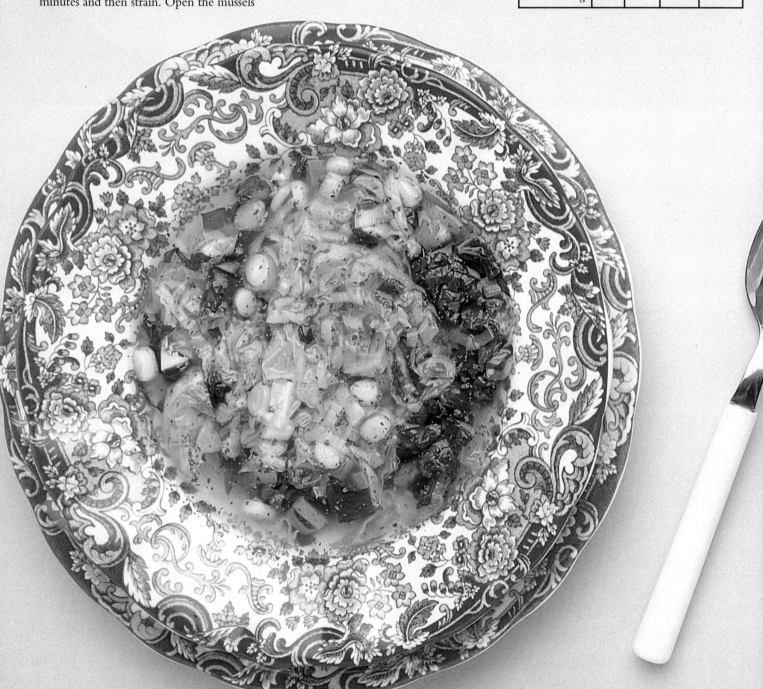

VEGETABLE SOUP

2 litres stock (home-made or cube)
100g leeks
200g lettuce
100g spinach
100g green beans
salt
2 tablespoons chopped, fresh mint

Clean the leeks and slice finely. Clean the lettuce and green beans and cut into strips. Clean the spinach and shred. Cook all the ingredients in the stock for 30 minutes. Season with the salt and mint.

	Cal.	Pro.	Fat	Carbo.
Per Serving	27	2.2	0.3	4.2

CHICKEN SOUP

1 litre stock (home-made or cube)
100g chicken breast
1 egg
50g Parma ham
1 tablespoon sherry

Pre-cooked chicken breast can be used, or, alternatively, fresh chicken can be boiled in the soup stock. Chop the cooked chicken into fine slivers. Cook the egg for 12 minutes, peel and chop. Chop the Parma ham into fine strips. Heat the stock with all the ingredients and add the sherry just before serving.

	Cal.	Pro.	Fat	Carbo.
Per Serving	103	8.2	7.8	-

TRADITIONAL BROTH

200g beef
250g chicken
1 onion
2 carrots
2 litres water
parsley

Place all the ingredients in cold water and bring to the boil. Then simmer for 3 hours (or 1½ hours in a pressure cooker). Strain and leave the liquid to cool completely.

When cold, skim off all the fat which will have solidified on the surface of the broth. Once this is done, the calorific value of the broth will be minimal (about 10 calories per person).

This broth can be made into a soup by adding:

Pasta   – 20g per person 72 cal.
Rice   – 20g per person 73 cal.
Vegetables – 100g per person 30 cal.

Left: Vegetable soup
Below: Traditional broth

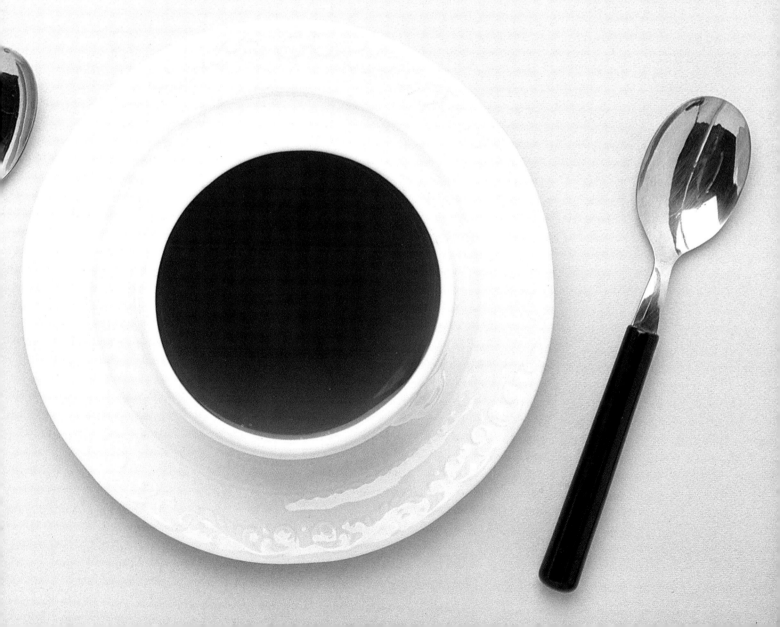

CURRY CREAM SOUP

1 litre stock (home-made or cube)
400g onion, sliced
20g cornflour
20g butter
250ml milk
100g apple, chopped
20g grated coconut
1 teaspoon curry powder
salt

Simmer the onion, apple and grated coconut in the stock for 15 minutes. Liquidize in a blender or food processor.

Dissolve the cornflour in the milk and add the onion–apple mixture, stirring well.

Heat until the mixture thickens, then continue to cook for a few minutes. Season with the curry powder and salt. Take off the heat and add the butter before serving.

This soup can also be served cold.

	Cal.	Pro.	Fat	Carbo.
Per Serving	113	3	7.15	9.2

CREAM OF TOMATO SOUP

500g tomatoes
100g celery
100g potato
100g onion
100g carrot
20g (2 tablespoons) flour
1 clove garlic, chopped
100ml brandy
thyme
salt & pepper

Simmer the chopped tomato, celery, carrot, potato, onion and clove of garlic in a litre of water for 25 minutes.

Liquidize in a blender or food processor. Add the flour mixed with the brandy and heat until it thickens slightly, stirring all the time.

Season according to taste with a little fresh, chopped thyme and salt and pepper.

	Cal.	Pro.	Fat	Carbo.
Per Serving	109	4	2.1	15.2

CREAM OF ENDIVE SOUP

500g endives, washed and chopped
100g potato, cubed
200g onion, chopped
1 clove garlic, chopped
100ml milk
100ml cream
40g bread, thinly sliced
nutmeg and salt

Place the onion, potato, endives and garlic in a pan with approximately 1 litre of water. Bring to the boil and simmer for about 20 minutes.

Liquidize in a food processor or blender. Add the cream and milk and season with nutmeg and salt. Serve with slices of toast.

	Cal.	Pro.	Fat	Carbo.
Per Serving	187	4.9	7.3	19.8

Top: Cream of Tomato Soup
Bottom: Curry Cream Soup

VEGETABLES AND SALADS

These are foods with a high vitamin and mineral content and which also provide undigestable vegetable fibre - cellulose. Cellulose has no calorific value, but gives the sensation of being full and promotes healthy digestion. The high calorific value of a plate of vegetables or salad comes from the oil dressing - for example:

1 tablespoon of olive oil   - 90 calories
1 portion of lettuce (50g)   - 8 calories
1 portion of cooked spinach (250g) - 50 calories

Therefore the quantity of oil or butter used to garnish vegetables should be kept to a minimum. Vinegar, lemon, garlic and onion have a very low calorific value and can also be used very effectively as a garnish or dressing. Some vegetables can be cooked in a stock to give them a particular flavour without increasing the calorific value, provided that the stock is fat free (see soups).

All the salad recipes listed on the following pages include low calory dressings.

CAULIFLOWER VINAIGRETTE

Serves 4

1 kg cauliflower
20g gherkins
20g capers
50g olives
20g sweet pepper
1 egg-white
4 anchovies
100g tomato
1 cup yoghurt
2 tablespoons olive oil
salt and lemon

Clean the cauliflower, break into florets and cook in boiling water with salt and lemon, taking care that the florets do not break up, then drain.

Prepare the vinaigrette by chopping the gherkins, anchovies, capers, olives and sweet pepper, and mixing together with the egg white. Wash the anchovies before chopping.

Scald the tomato in hot water to remove the skin, then remove the seeds as well and chop. Mix with the olive oil and yoghurt and add salt to taste. Mix well with the other ingredients (caper and anchovy mixture), cover the cauliflower with the vinaigrette and serve cold.

The yoghurt can be substituted by 1 tablespoon of vinegar and 2 of water.

	Cal.	Pro.	Fat	Carbo.
Per Serving	195	9.9	10	15.4

COURGETTES WITH CHEESE

Serves 4

1 kg courgettes
300g onion
100ml milk
100ml single cream
40g Roquefort cheese
Salt and white pepper

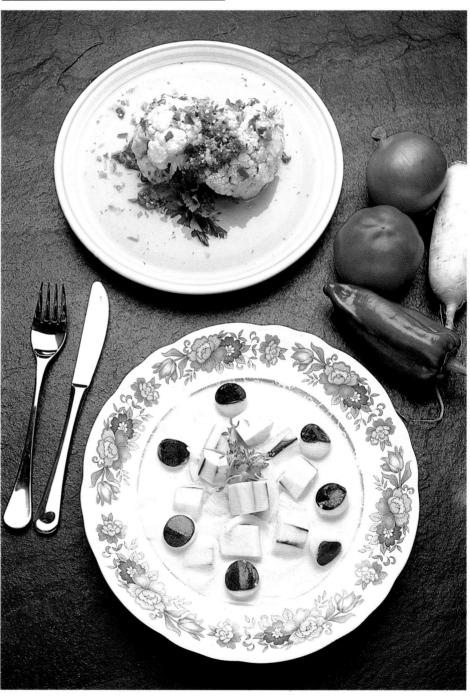

Top: Cauliflower Vinaigrette
Bottom: Courgettes with Cheese

Cut the onion into strips and cook in a little water until very soft. Then add the cleaned and diced courgettes and cook in their juices and the remainder of the water, stirring all the time. Add more water if necessary.

Mix the milk, water and cheese and season with salt and pepper.

When the courgettes are soft add the cheese sauce, heat gently for a short time and serve in a deep dish.

	Cal.	Pro.	Fat	Carbo.
Per Serving	187	5.2	9.3	-

ROQUEFORT DRESSING

2 egg whites
25g Roquefort cheese
100ml milk
50ml olive oil

Put all the ingredients in a liquidizer or food processor and blend well until you have a smooth liquid.

Use as a sauce or dressing.

	Cal.	Pro.	Fat	Carbo.
Total	547	11.9	53	2
1 tbsp	23	0.5	2.3	-

SWEET AND SOUR CABBAGE

Serves 4

1 kg cabbage
1/2 kg onion
10g butter
2 tablespoons olive oil
1 tablespoon sugar
1 tablespoon vinegar
1 teaspoon cumin seeds
salt

Clean the cabbage, finely chop and cook. When it is just cooked, drain thoroughly. Crush the cumin seeds with the salt, and mix the vinegar with the oil and then mix both with the drained cabbage.

Peel the onions, chop into fine strips and cook in a little water. When well-cooked, drain and add the butter, sugar and stir a little until the onions are golden.

Place half the cabbage in a bowl, cover with the onion mixture and top with the rest of the cabbage.

	Cal.	Pro.	Fat	Carbo.
Per Serving	163	5	5	26

MELON SALAD

Serves 4

1 kg cabbage
100g raisins
400g melon
200g carrot

This salad can be served with cream dressing, pepper dressing or traditional dressing.

Soak the raisins in water for 30 minutes. Clean the cabbage and slice into very fine strips. Chop the melon into small squares. Grate the carrot finely. Mix all the ingredients together, add the desired dressing and let it marinate for some time to develop the full flavour of the dressing. Serve cold.

	Cal.	Pro.	Fat	Carbo.
Per Serving	201	5.9	0.6	43

SIMPLE SALAD

800g cucumber
1 sprig mint
400g new potatoes
traditional or yoghurt dressing

Wash the potatoes and cook with their skins in salted water. Let them cool, then peel them and cut into slices. Peel the cucumber and cut into fine slices. Separate the leaves from the mint stalk.

Layer the potatoes and cucumber in a serving dish, sprinkle over the mint leaves and cover with the dressing. Leave to marinate for at least 30 minutes.

	Cal.	Pro.	Fat	Carbo.
Per Serving	117	3.6	0.	25+dressing

SALAD WITH PALM HEARTS

1/2 kg palm hearts (tinned)
250g mushrooms
250g carrots
juice of 2 lemons
50 ml olive oil
1 tablespoon fresh parsley, chopped
1 tablespoon fresh tarragon, chopped
pepper & salt

Clean the mushrooms and cut off the stalks. Put them in the lemon juice so that they don't become brown.

Peel the carrot, grate very finely and add to the mushrooms. Chop the palm hearts

into large slices. Add to the mushrooms and carrots. Blend together the oil, salt, parsley, tarragon and pepper. Pour this mixture onto the salad and leave for at least 30 minutes to develop the full taste. Serve at room temperature.

	Cal.	Pro.	Fat	Carbo.
Per Serving	191	3.5	10.7	20.2

TOMATO SALAD

Serves 4

800g tomatoes
800g potatoes
400g carrots
Mint
traditional or cream dressing

Scald the tomatoes and peel. Cut into large slices. Wash the potatoes and cook in salted water. Let them cool, then peel and cut into slices. Peel and finely grate the carrots. Chop up the mint. Mix all the ingredients together. Cover with the dressing and leave to marinate for at least 30 minutes.

Serve cold.

	Cal.	Pro.	Fat	Carbo.
Per Serving	158	5.1	0.9	36.2

Top: Tomato Salad
Bottom: Simple Salad

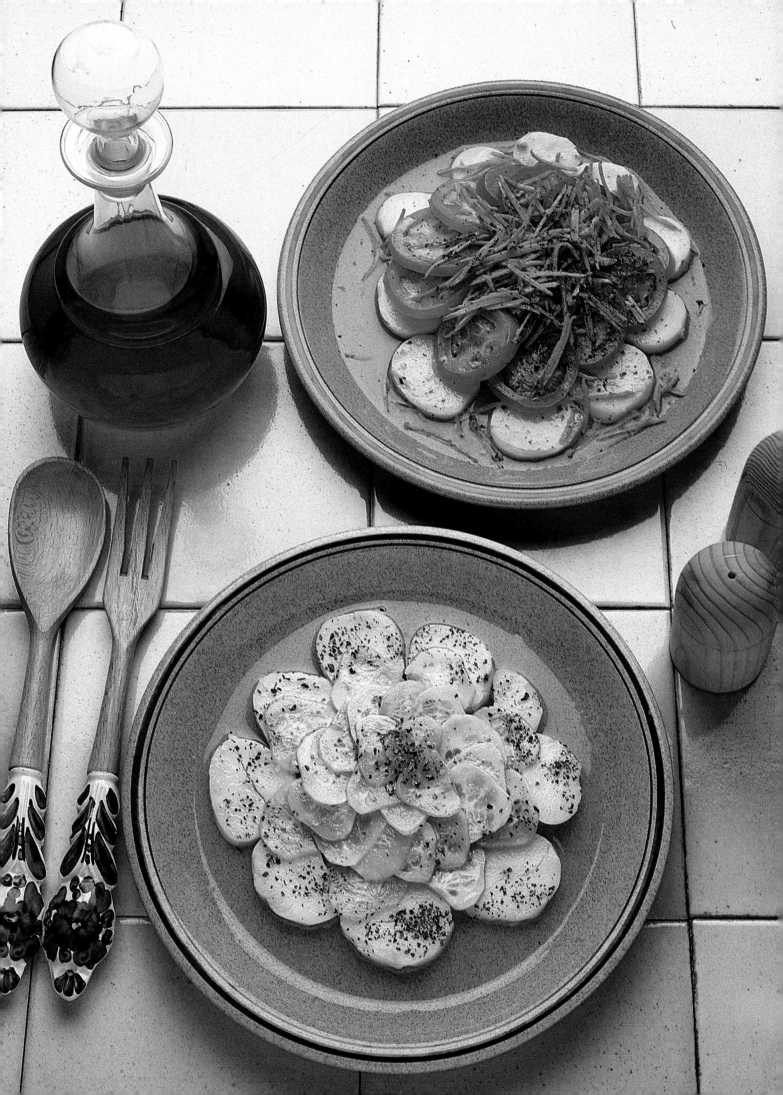

CARROTS IN CREAM

Serves 4

800g carrots
1/2 litre stock
100ml single cream
2 egg yolks
1 tablespoon chopped parsley
salt

Peel and slice the carrots and simmer in the stock until they are cooked and the stock has reduced to a few spoonfuls.

Place the carrots in an ovenproof dish and mix the reduced stock with the single cream, egg yolks and parsley. Season. Pour the sauce over the carrots, and heat for a few minutes in the oven but do not allow to bubble or boil.

	Cal.	Pro.	Fat	Carbo.
Per Serving	187	5.2	9.3	-

MIXED SALAD

Serves 4

1 lettuce
1/2 kg carrots
1/4 kg cucumber
2 apples
1/4 kg red cabbage
French dressing or yoghurt

Wash the lettuce and red cabbage and chop finely. Clean and grate the carrots. Peel and slice the cucumber. Peel the apples and cut into thin strips.

Mix all the ingredientts together and add the dressing. Leave to marinate for 30 minutes. Serve cold.

	Cal.	Pro.	Fat	Carbo.
Per Serving	51	1.6	0.4	*10+dressing*

Left: Carrots in cream
Right: Mixed salad

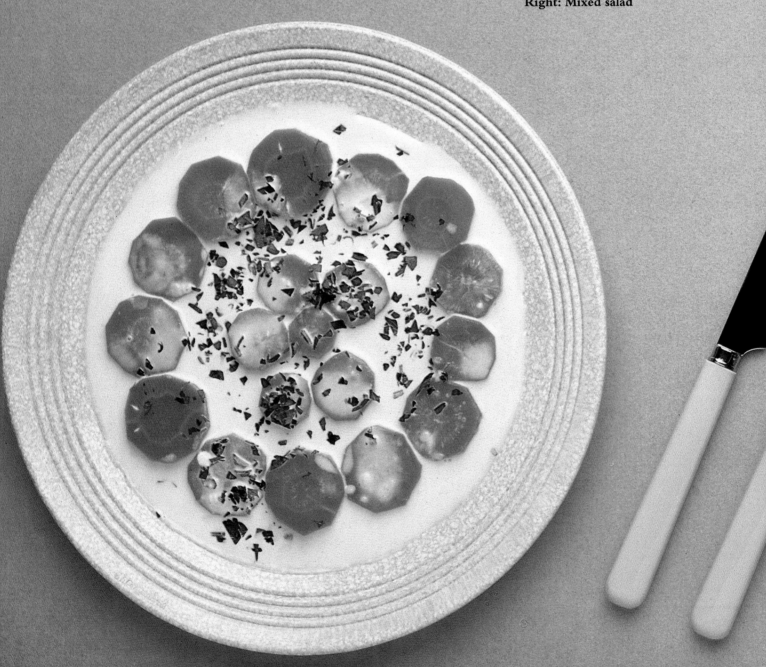

INSTANT SALAD

500g endives
Roquefort sauce (1 serving)

Wash the endives and chop into large pieces.
   Make the Roquefort sauce following the recipe on page 18.
   Cover the endives with the sauce and serve cold.

	Cal.	Pro.	Fat	Carbo.
Per Serving	200	4.4	13.3	47

SIMPLE DRESSING

¹/₂ cup oil
50 ml vinegar
1 tablespoon Worcester sauce
1 teaspoon mustard
salt

Blend all the ingredients together, mixing in the oil last, a little at a time.

	Cal.	Pro.	Fat	Carbo.
Total	900	-	100	-
Per Serving	60	-	6.6	-

PEPPER DRESSING

¹/₂ cup olive oil
juice of 1 lemon
1 teaspoon pepper
cumin seeds and salt

Heat the oil for a short time in a frying pan, add the pepper and when it starts to heat up, add the lemon juice, then remove the pan from the heat.
   Pour into a liquidizer, add the cumin and the salt and mix well. Use immediately.

	Cal.	Pro.	Fat	Carbo.
Total	924	0.4	100	5.7
Per Tbsp	61	-	6.6	0.3

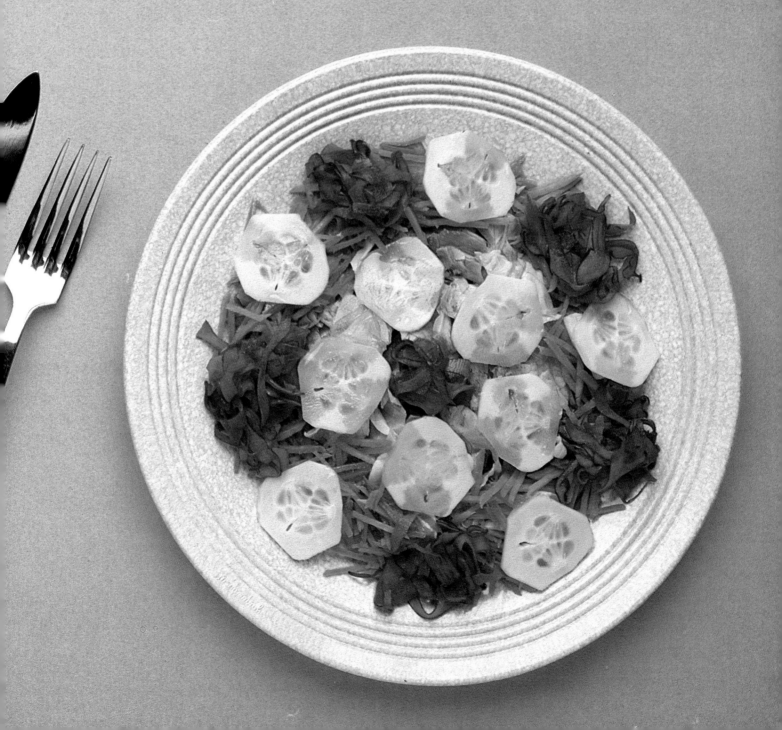

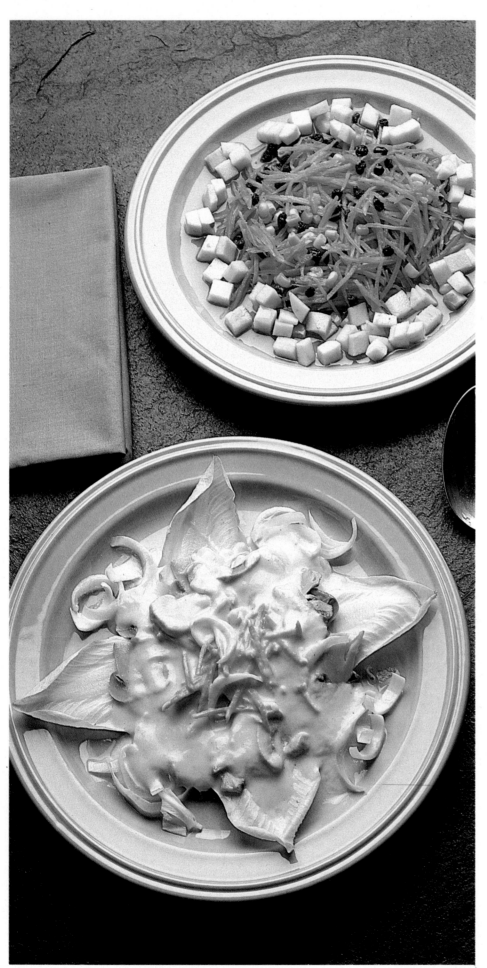

AMERICAN SALAD

Serves 4

800g carrots
¹/₂ kg tin sweetcorn
500g butter
juice of 3 oranges
50g currants
yoghurt dressing, cream, egg white or traditional dressing

Soak the currants in water for 30 minutes. Peel and finely slice the carrot and leave to soak in the orange juice for an hour to absorb the taste. Then add the drained currants, sweetcorn and diced apple. Add your dressing of choice and serve cold.

	Cal.	Pro.	Fat	Carbo.
Per Serving	285	3.1	1	65.9+*dressing*

SALAD WITH CHEESE

Serves 4

250g endives
100g Roquefort cheese
400g carrots
200g mushrooms
juice of 1 lemon
juice of 1 orange
50ml olive oil
pepper and salt

Peel and grate the carrots and leave to marinate in the orange juice for 1 hour.
  Clean the mushrooms, cutting off the stalks and marinate in the lemon juice.
  Place the cheese and the olive oil in a blender or liquidizer and mix well. Add the juice from the carrots and the mushrooms and season. Chop the endives, mix with the mushrooms and carrots and cover with the cheese dressing. Let it stand for a short time before serving.

	Cal.	Pro.	Fat	Carbo.
Per Serving	258	5.6	19.9	14.1

Left, top: American Salad
Left, bottom: Salad with Cheese
Opposite, top: Stuffed Peppers (recipe on page 24)
Opposite, bottom: Spinach with Prawns & Rice (recipe on page 24)

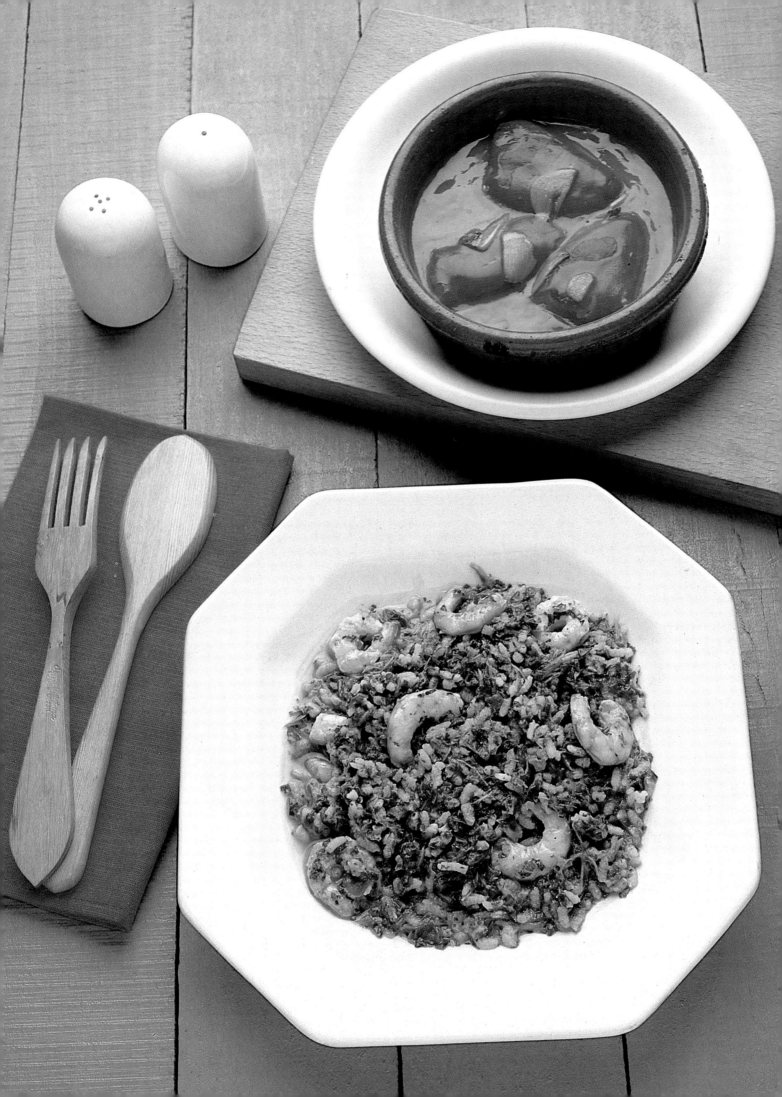

STUFFED PEPPERS

Serves 4

8 red peppers, with core and seeds removed
200g cooked and mashed potato
16 prawns
100g hake, chopped
2 tablespoons olive oil
2 cloves garlic, chopped
100ml white wine
rosemary and salt

Gently re-heat the cooked, mashed potato, and add the raw hake and the prawns. Season with salt and rosemary.

Stuff the peppers with this mixture and place in an ovenproof dish.

Put the oil in a frying pan and brown the garlic. Add all of the white wine and let it reduce a little. Add a few spoonfuls of water and pour this mixture over the peppers in the ovenproof dish. Bake in the oven at a moderate heat for 30-40 minutes.

	Cal.	Pro.	Fat	Carbo.
Per Serving	158	6	9.9	13.2

SPINACH WITH PRAWNS AND RICE

Serves 4

1 kg spinach
80g rice
20 prawns
2 cloves garlic, chopped
3 tablespoons olive oil
juice of 1 lemon
salt

Clean the spinach, remove the stalks and cook. Drain and chop. You can use frozen spinach if preferred.

Peel the prawns and make about ½ litre of stock with the shells. Fry the garlic in the oil until golden and then sauté the rice. Mix well and add the chopped spinach. Add prawn stock to the rice and cook. When the stock is boiling add the lemon juice, salt and prawns. Add more stock if necessary during the cooking time.

	Cal.	Pro.	Fat	Carbo.
Per Serving	220	11	8.6	24

EGG WHITE DRESSING

2 egg whites
1 tablespoon mustard
100ml olive oil

Put the egg whites into a deep bowl and beat a little, add the mustard and then the olive oil a little at a time and mix well. It should remain fluid. Serve cold.

	Cal.	Pro.	Fat	Carbo.
Total	750	6.6	80	0.6
1 Tbsp	39	0.3	4.2	-

TRADITIONAL DRESSING

200 ml olive oil
50 ml vinegar
1 tablespoon chopped parsley
salt

Put all the ingredients into a blender or liquidizer. Mix well and use.

	Cal.	Pro.	Fat	Carbo.
Total	1.140	-	160	-
1 Tbsp	72	-	8	-

WINTER SALAD

Serves 4

1 kg cabbage
300g apple
100g rice
100g sweetcorn
egg white, traditional, pepper or yoghurt dressing

Wash the cabbage and chop finely.

Cook the rice in plenty of salted water for 20 minutes, stirring frequently. Drain and cool.

Peel and dice the apple and put in water with a little lemon juice added if it is not going to be used immediately.

Mix together the cabbage, rice, apple and dressing and leave to marinate for at least 1 hour.

	Cal.	Pro.	Fat	Carbo.
Per Serving	287	6.4	1.7	61+dressing

GARDEN SALAD

Serves 4

500g artichokes
400g potatoes
200g gherkins
200g tomatoes
8 radishes
yoghurt, traditional, simple or pepper dressing

Prepare the artichokes, leaving just the hearts. Put them in a pan with cold water. Add a tablespoon of flour dissolved in a little water, and the flesh of a skinless, pipless lemon, so that the artichoke does not become bitter. Cook for 15-20 minutes. Then let the artichokes cool in the cooking water.

Cook the washed but unpeeled potatoes. After cooking, peel and dice. Slice the gherkins lengthways. Scald the tomatoes and peel them. Cut them into quite small slices.

Mix together all the ingredients.

Add the dressing and leave to marinate for 30 or 40 minutes and serve cold.

	Cal.	Pro.	Fat	Carbo.
Per Serving	177	4.7	0.5	24.2

Top: Winter Salad
Bottom: Garden Salad

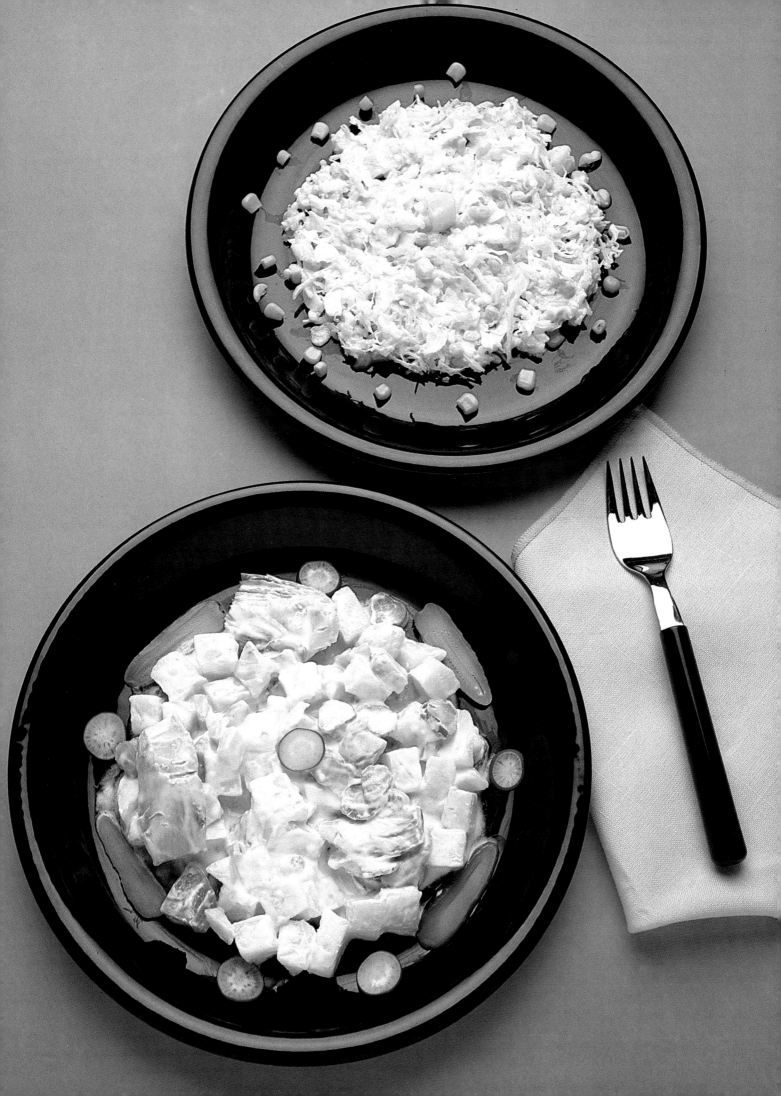

LEEKS IN WHITE SAUCE

Serves 4

800g leeks
2 tablespoons flour
30g butter
3 cloves garlic, chopped
30g ground almonds
salt and pepper

Clean the leeks and cook whole, reserving the cooking water.

Fry the garlic in the butter until golden and then add the flour. Sauté, then add the stock from the leeks a little at a time, stirring, until the flour and liquid are well blended. Add the ground almonds and cook until the sauce thickens.

When it is ready, season with salt and pepper and pour over the leeks.

	Cal.	Pro.	Fat	Carbo.
Per Serving	175	4.1	9	18

GREEN BEANS WITH PEPPERS

Serves 4

800g green beans
500g red peppers
4 tablespoons olive oil

Below: Leeks in White Sauce
Right: Aranjuez Salad

2 cloves garlic, chopped
2 tablespoons chopped parsley
salt

Top and tail the beans, wash them and cook in boiling salted water for about 10 minutes. Roast the red peppers in the oven or under the grill until the skin is black and blistered, then peel them and cut

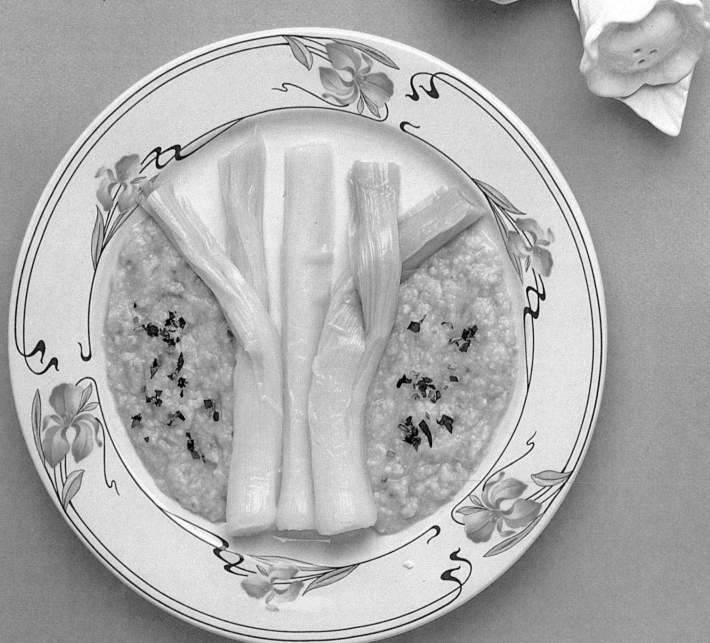

into strips. Fry the garlic in the olive oil and, when golden, add the chopped parsley and the roast peppers. Add the green beans, cooked and drained. Stir well and serve hot.

	Cal.	Pro.	Fat	Carbo.
Per Serving	200	6.5	10.6	19.6

ARANJUEZ SALAD

Serves 4

500g asparagus
1 lettuce (approx. 200g)
300g potatoes
traditional, egg white or pepper dressing

Clean the asparagus removing the fibrous parts of the stalks. Cook the asparagus in salted water, ensuring it is constantly covered in water and that it cooks slowly so that the tips do not break off. Let it cool in the cooking water.

Clean and shred the lettuce and leave to soak in cold water until ready to use.

Cook the washed but unpeeled potatoes, then peel and cut into slices. Cover a plate with a layer of potatoes, then add a layer of well drained lettuce, then place the asparagus on top. Pour over the dressing and leave to marinate for at least 30 minutes for the taste to develop.

Serve cold.

	Cal.	Pro.	Fat	Carbo.
Per Serving	120	4.7	0.5	24.2+*dressing*

SOYA BEAN SALAD

Serves 4

1/2 kg tin of soya bean shoots
2 bunches watercress
500g carrots
yoghurt or traditional dressing

Clean the watercress retaining only the leaves. Chop up the soya bean shoots. Clean and finely grate the carrot. Combine the ingredients and pour over the dressing. Leave for 15-20 minutes and serve cold.

	Cal.	Pro.	Fat	Carbo.
Per Serving	125	7.1	1.6.	21+*dressing*

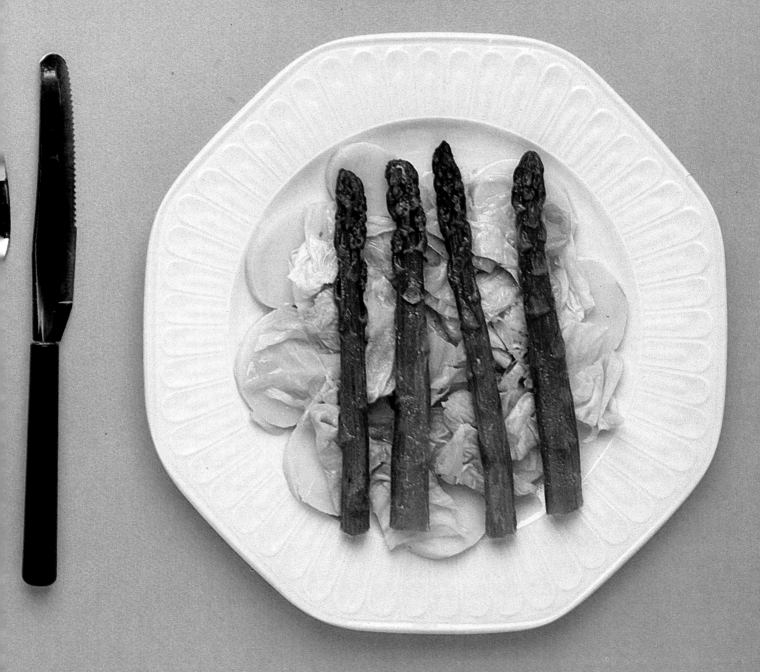

ARTICHOKES WITH SOFT CHEESE

Serves 4

4 medium sized artichokes
200g soft cheese
200g onions
20g butter
1 tablespoon cornflour
1/2 litre stock
1 lemon
Salt

Clean the artichokes by removing the hard leaves and the hairy centres from inside. Rub them with lemon and cook in water with salt and lemon juice. When cooked, drain and then stuff with the soft cheese and place in an ovenproof dish.

Cook the chopped onion in the stock and when it is soft add the butter and the cornflour dissolved in a little cold milk. Cook the sauce, then sieve and cover the artichokes with it.

Put the dish in a moderate oven for a few minutes until the cheese has melted.

	Cal.	Pro.	Fat	Carbo.
Per Serving	233	11.7	8.7	27

ENDIVES AU GRATIN

Serves 4

8 endives
50g York ham
100g grated cheese
100ml single cream
100ml milk
1 egg yolk

Wash the endives and cook them whole, taking care that they do not break up. Drain well and place in an ovenproof dish. Mix together the cream, milk and egg yolk and cover the endives with the mixture. Cut the ham into fine strips and place on the endives. Sprinkle with the grated cheese and brown in the oven.

	Cal.	Pro.	Fat	Carbo.
Per Serving	174	6.1	12.6	0.9

BEETROOT SALAD

Serves 4

400g beetroot
500g apple
300g melon
200g turnip
traditional or cream dressing

Cook the beetroot in cold water with salt – do not peel or cut at this stage. When cooked, drain, peel and cut into large cubes. Peel and dice the apple. Leave it in cold water with lemon juice to prevent it from turning brown. Dice the melon. Finely dice or grate the turnip.

Mix the ingredients together and add one of the suggested dressings; leave to stand for a while so that the taste develops.

	Cal.	Pro.	Fat	Carbo.
Per Serving	151	3.1	0.8	32+dressing

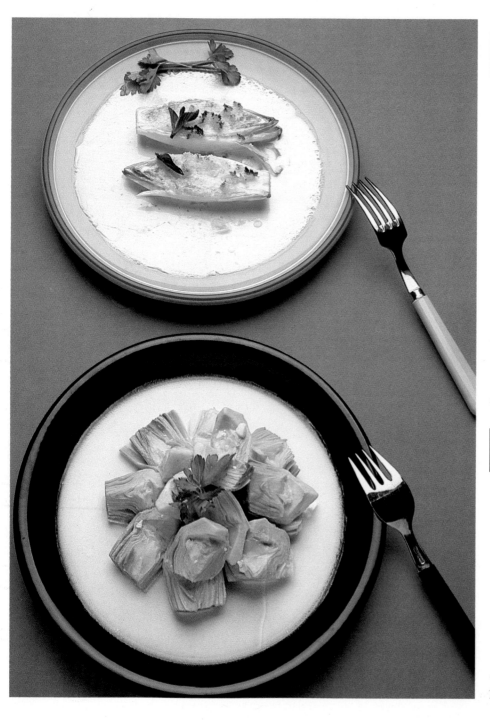

Top: Endives au Gratin
Bottom: Artichokes with Soft Cheese

CREAM DRESSING

200ml single cream
50ml olive oil
juice of 1 lemon
1 tablespoon chopped parsley
pepper and salt

Lightly whip the cream and add the olive oil a little at a time; then mix in the lemon juice, parsley, salt and pepper. Blend together and keep cool prior to serving.

	Cal.	Pro.	Fat	Carbo.
Total	1026	5	87.6	13.9
1 Tbsp	41	0.26	3.5	0.5

STUFFED LETTUCE

Serves 4

2 large lettuces
400g mushrooms, slices
100g onions, finely chopped
2 tablespoons breadcrumbs
20g butter
Meat stock (fat free)
juice of ½ lemon
salt

Wash the lettuces, remove the outer leaves and cook whole in the stock. Drain and cut in half lengthways. Cook the mushrooms and onion in water with the salt and lemon juice. Drain.

Stuff the lettuce halves with the mushrooms and onions, folding them over to form a parcel, then place them in an ovenproof dish, spooning over a little of the stock used during cooking.

Sprinkle with breadcrumbs and butter and brown in the oven.

	Cal.	Pro.	Fat	Carbo.
Per Serving	120	10	5.5	9

VEGETABLE ROAST

Serves 4

4 aubergines, each weighing
   approximately 200g
2 large tomatoes
4 medium sized potatoes
4 red peppers
4 tablespoons olive oil
salt

Wipe the aubergines with a cloth and roast in the oven until soft and wrinkled (approximately an hour). Clean the tomatoes, cut in half and roast. Wash the potatoes, wrap each one in foil and bake until soft. Clean the peppers and roast.

Peel the aubergines and peppers (both peel more easily if they are covered with a cloth for a short time after they are roasted) and slice. Take the potatoes from the foil.

Arrange the vegetables in groups and season, then dress with the four tablespoons of oil.

	Cal.	Pro.	Fat	Carbo.
Per Serving	270	11	6	37

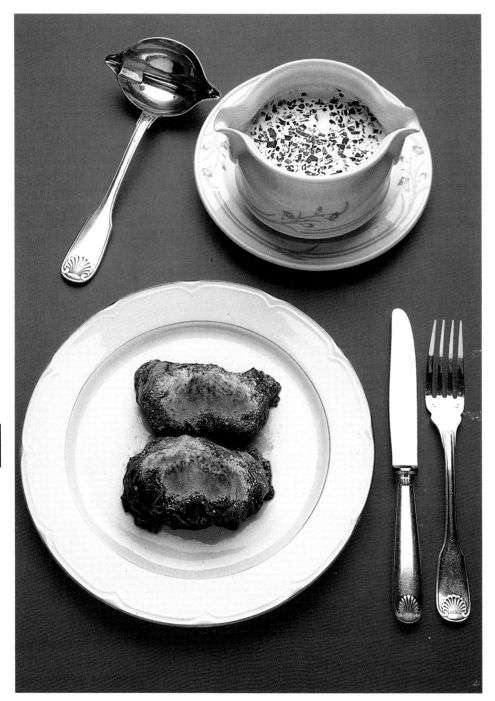

Top: Cream Dressing
Bottom: Stuffed Lettuce

YOGHURT DRESSING

1 small tub of natural yoghurt
¹/2 dl olive oil
juice of 1 lemon
pepper and salt

Mix all the ingredients in a blender or liquidizer. Taste and season.

	Cal.	Pro.	Fat	Carbo.
Total	444	5.2	44	7
1 Tbsp	34	0.4	33	0.5

VEGETABLE STEW

Serves 4

200g carrots
500g green beans
200g silver-beet leaves
300g artichokes
200g onions
2 cloves garlic, chopped
1 slice bread
olive oil
salt

Cook the vegetables separately: chop the carrots into batons, dice the green beans, halve the artichokes and finely slice the silver-beet leaves.

Cook the finely chopped onion in a small amount of water or stock, so that when cooked there is only a little liquid. In a little oil, fry the garlic cloves without burning, then put them to one side in a mortar dish. Also fry the bread and add to the garlic. Crush them with a little salt. Dissolve them in the stock produced from cooking either the green beans or carrots. Then in an earthenware dish place the vegetables mixed with the cooked onion. Add the crushed garlic, bread and stock mixture and some more stock if necessary. Cook all the ingredients for a few minutes. The dish can be garnished with asparagus if desired.

	Cal.	Pro.	Fat	Carbo.
Per Serving	192	7.5	32	33.4

CATALAN SALAD

Serves 4

500g mushrooms
150g rice
100g tinned sweetcorn
small bunch of parsley
salt & pepper
lemon juice
egg white dressing

Cook the rice in plenty of salted water for about 20 minutes. Drain, rinse with cold water and put aside.

Clean the mushrooms, chop off the stalks and cover with a little lemon juice to avoid browning. Drain the sweetcorn and chop the parsley. Mix all the ingredients together and serve cool.

	Cal.	Pro.	Fat	Carbo.
Per Serving	252	10	0.4	52+dressing

POMEGRANATE SALAD

Serves 4

1 endive
2 pomegranates
250g carrots
2 cloves garlic, chopped
¹/2 dl olive oil
¹/2 dl vinegar
pepper and salt

Wash the endive, slice finely and place in cold water. Clean and deseed the pomegranates. Clean and grate the carrots. Add the ingredients together and season; also add a little vinegar. Put the oil in a frying pan and fry the finely chopped garlic. When golden add to the salad, tossing well. Leave to stand for about 15 minutes to achieve the best taste.

Any other dressings can be added, according to taste.

	Cal.	Pro.	Fat	Carbo.
Per Serving	157	2.4	103	13.5+dressing

SILVER-BEET LEAVES WITH COCKLES

Serves 4

800g silver-beet stalks
300g carrots, sliced and cooked
200g onions
1 small tin cockles
1 dl white wine
salt
juice of ¹/2 lemon
2 tablespoons chopped parsley
olive oil

Clean the silver-beet stalks, removing any fibrous strands and cut them into 5cm pieces. Cook in water with salt and lemon. Fry the onion in a little oil. When cooked, drain away the oil, leaving the onion in the pan. Add the chopped parsley and the cooked carrot. Add the wine and allow to reduce. Add the cockles including the juice from the tin.

Mix the silver-beet stalks with the fried mixture and cook everything for a few minutes, adding water or stock if necessary.

	Cal.	Pro.	Fat	Carbo.
Per Serving	151	7.8	3.2	22.7

Top: Vegetable Stew
Bottom: Pomegranate Salad

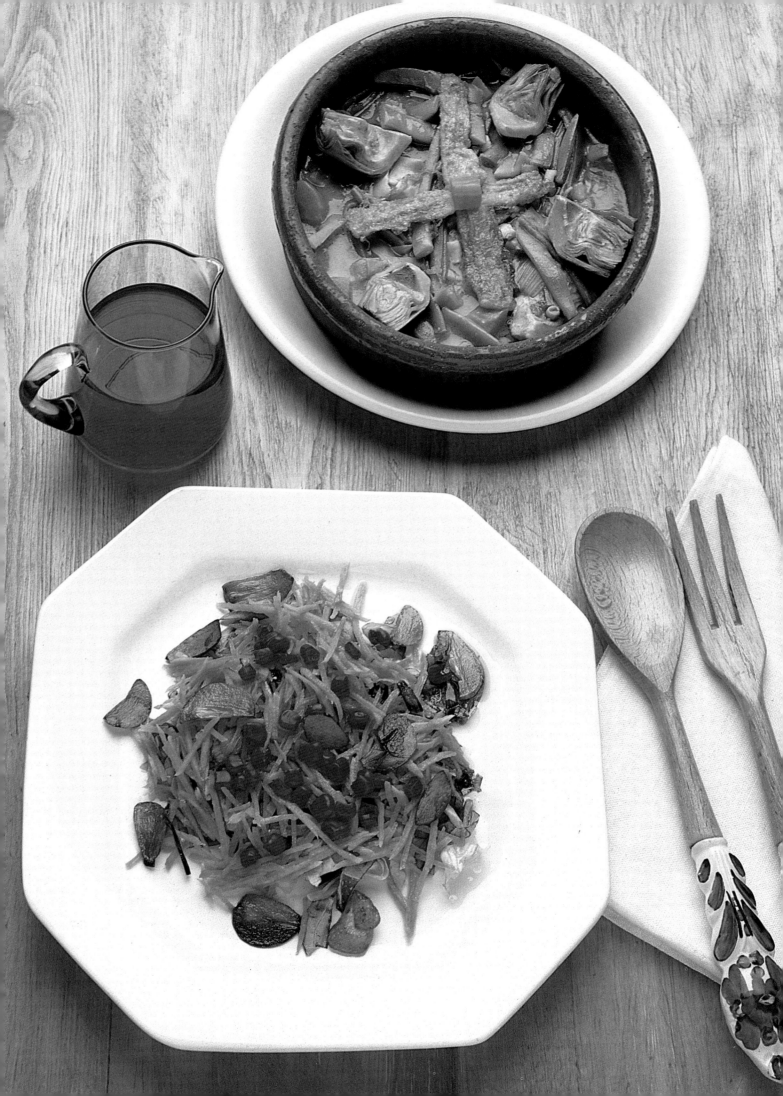

SILVER-BEET WITH CHICKPEAS

Serves 4

1 kg silver-beet
250g (80g uncooked) chickpeas
200g onion, chopped
1 clove garlic
1 tablespoon paprika
olive oil
salt
vinegar

Fry the onion in a little olive oil, and, when cooked, carefully drain away all of the oil. Add the finely chopped garlic, cook quickly until golden; add the paprika and a little water or stock so it does not burn, and then add a little vinegar.

Wash and chop the silver-beet and cook in salted water.

If you are using uncooked chickpeas, simmer them in water for about 45 minutes, after having soaked them in water overnight.

Mix the fried ingredients with the silver-beet and chickpeas, and if necessary add a little stock or cooking water from the chickpeas, although the mixture should not resemble a soup.

	Cal.	Pro.	Fat	Carbo.
Per Serving	183	10.7	4	26

Left: Silver-beet with Chickpeas
Right: Silver-beet leaves with Cockles (recipe on page 30)

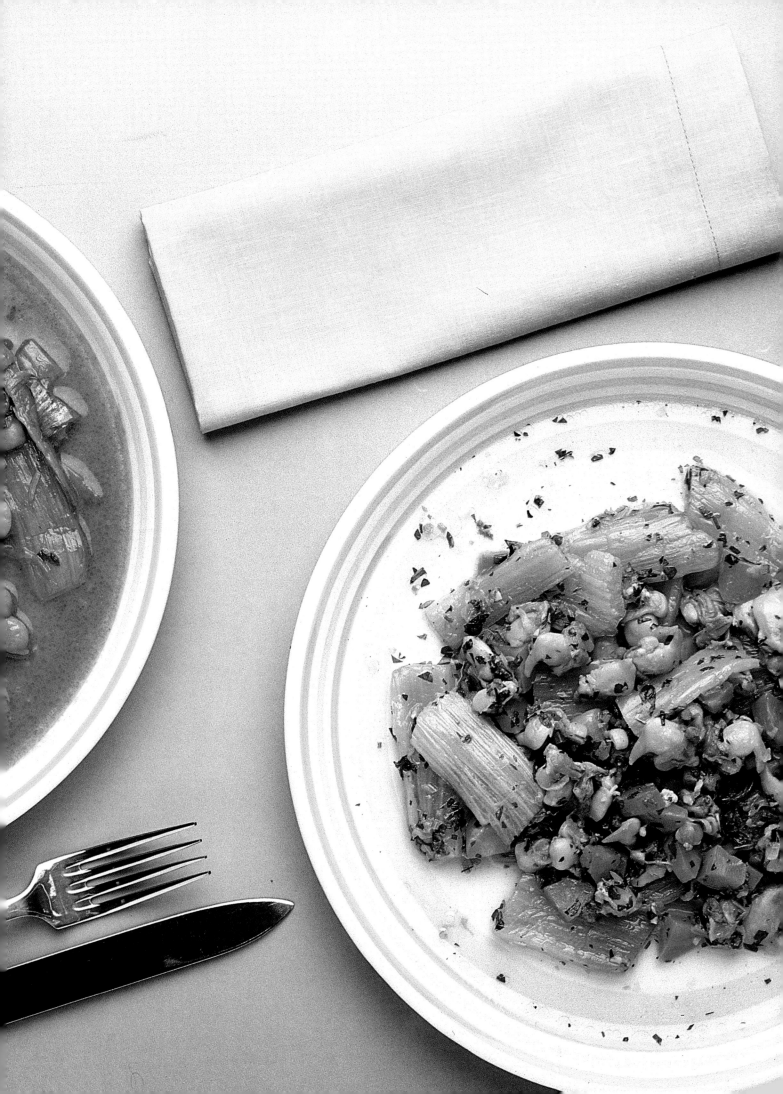

EGGS

One egg contains 76 calories and approximately 6 grammes of high biological value protein. There is no reason why eggs cannot be included in diets for slimmers to add variety to the diet, provided that low-fat cooking methods are used and they are combined with low energy-value ingredients.

EGGS WITH ASPARAGUS AND SPINACH

Serves 4

4 eggs
400g spinach
12 spears asparagus
100g onion
20g butter
salt

The eggs can be poached in boiling water or fried with very little oil in a non-stick pan. Finely chop the onion and cook in a little water so that when it is cooked hardly any liquid remains; add the butter and the cleaned, stalk-free spinach (frozen spinach can be used). Sauté the spinach, adding a little water if necessary, and cook with the lid on so it cooks in its own juices.

Cook the asparagus until "al dente," and mix with the spinach.

Place the freshly cooked eggs on top of the spinach and asparagus mixture to serve.

	Cal.	Pro.	Fat	Carbo.
Per Serving	161	10	10	8

SPINACH AND PRAWN OMELETTE

Serves 4

4 eggs
400g spinach
100g onion
15 prawns
15g butter
1 clove garlic
Olive oil (minimum amount needed for a non-stick frying pan)

Cook the finely chopped onion in about half a glass of water; when cooked add the washed and stalk-free spinach (it can be frozen) and cook together, adding a little water if necessary.

Put the butter into a frying pan, add the chopped garlic and the prawns, stir and add the spinach and onion.

Make 4 round omelettes with the eggs and fill each with the spinach and prawn stuffing, handling them carefully as 1 egg omelettes break easily.

The prawns can be substituted by 100g of soft cheese which is mixed with the spinach just before filling the omelettes.

	Cal.	Pro.	Fat	Carbo.
Per Serving	145	10.7	8.8	6.2

FRIED EGGS WITH RICE

Serves 4

4 eggs
4 tomatoes
80g rice
1 tablespoon oil
1 clove garlic
1 teaspoon sugar
salt
1 tablespoon chopped oregano
1 tablespoon chopped parsley
juice of 1/2 lemon

Clean the tomatoes, cut in half and put them in a roasting tin after sprinkling with oregano, parsley and a pinch of sugar. Roast until very soft and season.

Fry the garlic then sauté the rice in 1 tablespoon of oil. Add double the volume of water or stock and the juice of half a lemon and cook until the rice is ready and the water absorbed. (You may have to add more water).

Fry the eggs in a non-stick frying pan. Serve each egg with 2 halves of roasted tomato and a portion of rice; you can use a mould to create a rice shape.

	Cal.	Pro.	Fat	Carbo.
Per Serving	198	8.7	8.7	20

SCRAMBLED EGGS ON TOAST

Serves 4

4 eggs
4 slices bread
400g mushrooms
100g tinned pimientos
20g butter
juice of 1/2 lemon
salt & pepper
parsley

Toast the bread. Sauté the mushrooms in the butter with salt and the lemon juice. When cooked, add the pimientos, chopped into small pieces and the eggs beaten with salt and pepper. Cook, stirring all the time. Divide the mixture between the 4 pieces of toast and sprinkle with parsley.

	Cal.	Pro.	Fat	Carbo.
Per Serving	209	12.7	10.4	16.8

BOILED EGG SALAD

Serves 4

4 eggs
400g tomatoes
400g roasted, skinned fresh peppers
* or pimientos*
3 tablespoons oil
1 tablespon freshly chopped parsley
salt

Cook the eggs for 12 minutes, peel and cut into slices. Scald the tomatoes in boiling water, then peel them and cut into slices. Chop the peppers into wide strips (if roasted, peel first). Mix everything together and garnish with the olive oil, salt and lots of chopped parsley.

	Cal.	Pro.	Fat	Carbo.
Per Serving	210	33.2	135	38.4

**Top: Scrambled Eggs on Toast
Bottom: Eggs with Asparagus and Spinach**

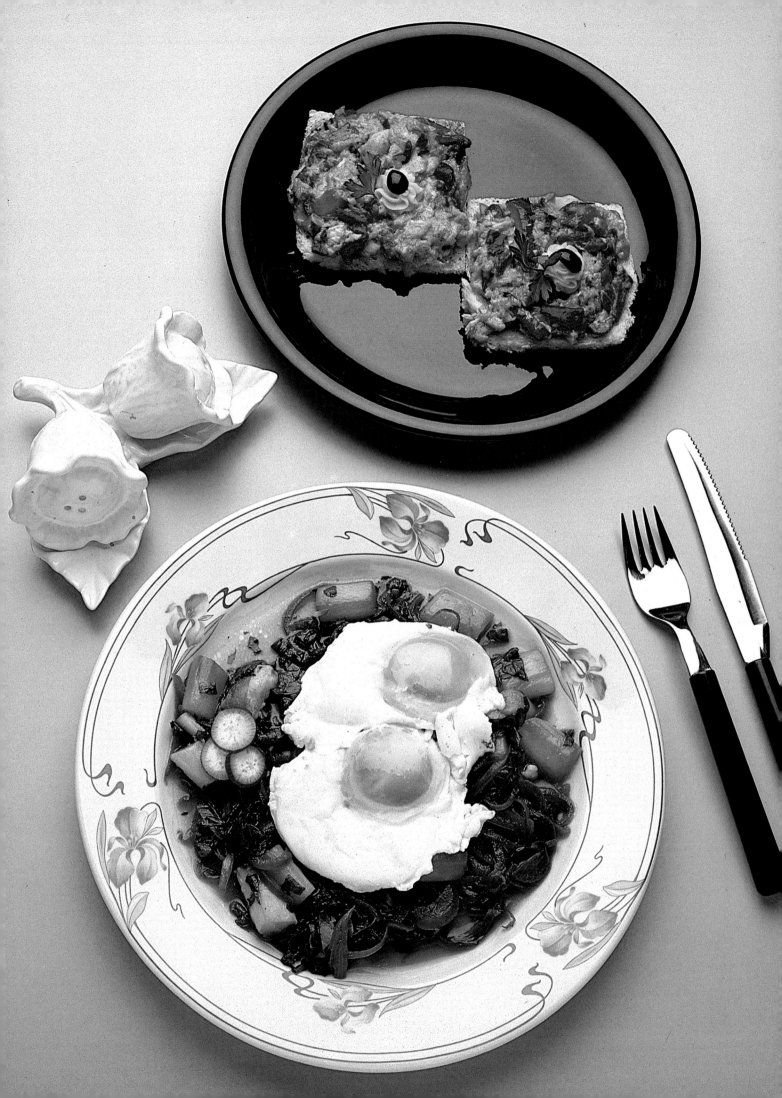

OMELETTE WITH ASPARAGUS

Serves 4

25 asparagus spears
4 eggs
1 slice bread
2 cloves garlic, chopped
1 tablespoon vinegar
olive oil
salt

Clean the asparagus and cook in a little water - place them horizontally in the pan, so they do not break.

In a little oil, fry the garlic cloves without burning and put aside in a mortar (dish). Fry the bread in the same oil and also add to the mortar. Crush the garlic and bread with a little salt and then dissolve the mixture in water used from cooking the asparagus and a little vinegar.

In a non-stick frying pan add a tiny amount of oil and then add beaten egg mixture so it covers the bottom. When half-cooked, add six asparagus spears, a few spoonfuls of the garlic and bread mixture and then fold the omelette over. Finish cooking, not allowing it to become too dry.

	Cal.	Pro.	Fat	Carbo.
Per Serving	*142*	*8.2*	*10.6*	*4.5*

EGGS SUNNYSIDE-UP

Serves 4

4 eggs
¹/₄ litre tomato juice (tinned)
400g green beans, cooked
100g Parma ham
12 asparagus tips

Divide the tomato juice between four individual dishes, and add the cooked green beans and chopped Parma ham. Put in the oven until the sauce boils.

Break the eggs over the hot sauce and garnish with the asparagus. Put the dish back in the oven and cook until the white of the egg is set; take care not to overcook as the yolk must remain soft.

	Cal.	Pro.	Fat	Carbo.
Per Serving	*214*	*14*	*12.9*	*10.5*

EGG MOULDS

Serves 4

4 eggs
400g mushrooms
1 lemon
1 dl white wine
1 clove garlic, chopped
2 tablespoons olive oil
butter to grease moulds

Clean the mushrooms and cook whole in water with the juice of half a lemon and some salt.

Fry the garlic in the oil until golden and add the cooked and drained mushrooms, the wine and the juice of half a lemon. Cook for a few minutes to reduce the wine.

Grease four individual flan moulds with butter. At the bottom place some mushrooms and the unbeaten egg. Cook in a bain-marie so the yolk does not harden.

Remove the mould and serve with the rest of the mushrooms.

	Cal.	Pro.	Fat	Carbo.
Per Serving	*147*	*10.1*	*10.9*	*3.3*

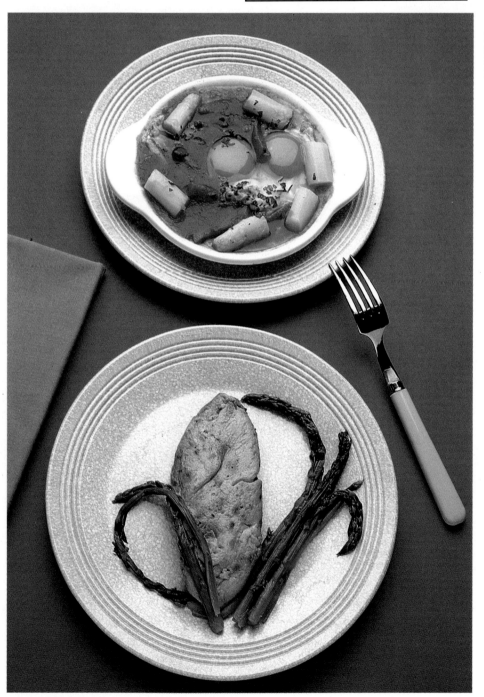

Left, top: Eggs Sunnyside-up
Left, bottom: Asparagus Omelette
Right, top: Fried Eggs with Rice
(recipe on page 34)
Right, bottom: Egg Moulds

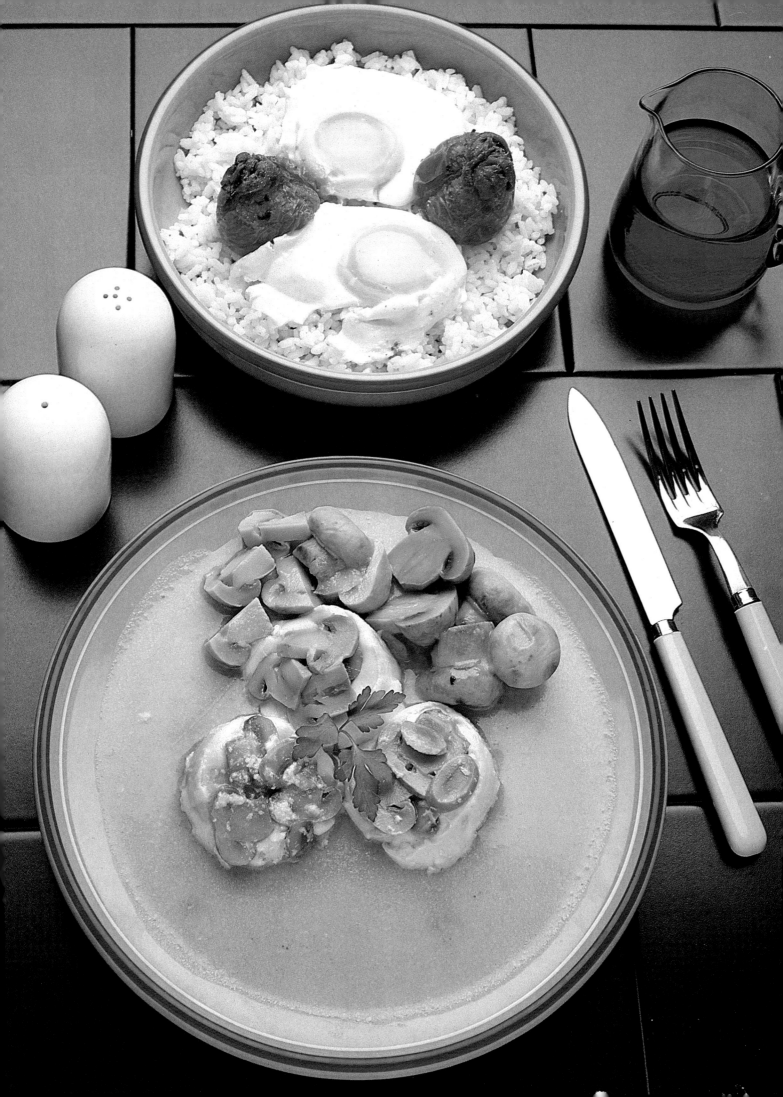

EGGS WITH MUSHROOM AND CHICKEN

Serves 4

4 eggs
100g roast chicken breast
50g Parma ham
400g mushrooms, sliced
100g onion, finely chopped
1/2 glass white wine
3 tablespoons olive oil
lemon juice
salt

Fry the onion in the oil until soft. Add the mushrooms and cook for a few minutes. Then add the ham and chicken, cut into large pieces.

Pour in the wine and cook for a few minutes to reduce. Season with salt and lemon juice.

Divide the sauce between four plates and put an egg on each one. Cook in the oven for a few minutes, making sure that the yolk does not become hard.

	Cal.	Pro.	Fat	Carbo.
Per Serving	*242*	*16*	*18*	*5.6*

EGGS WITH MASHED POTATO

Serves 4

4 eggs
100g soft cheese
10g Roquefort cheese
1/4 litre tomato juice
300g potato
1 dl milk for the mashed potato

Cook the eggs for 12 minutes until hard-boiled. Peel and cut in half lengthways and remove the yolks. Mix the yolks with the soft cheese and the Roquefort and 4 tablespoons of milk, then stuff each half of the egg with this mixture.

Boil the potatoes, add the rest of the milk and mash them. Place the eggs on a plate, surrounding them with piped mashed potato, and cover with a little hot tomato sauce, leaving the rest of the sauce in a jug.

The cheese can be substituted by anchovies, which should be washed to remove the oil.

	Cal.	Pro.	Fat	Carbo.
Per Serving	*225*	*11.2*	*10.4*	*20.2*

Left: Eggs with Mushroom and Chicken
Right: Eggs with Mashed Potato

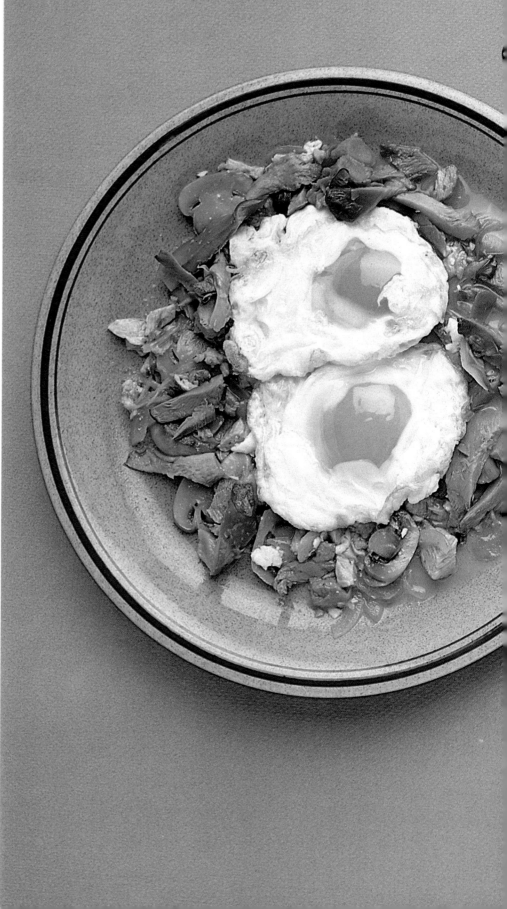

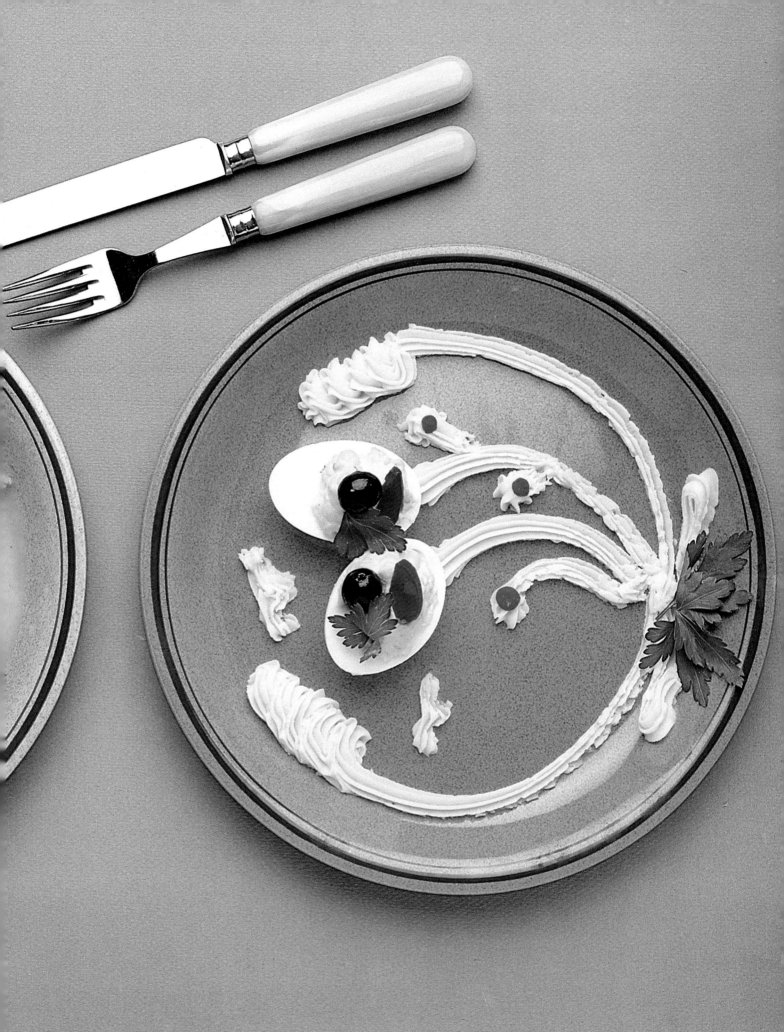

SEAFOOD

Fish contains protein of high biological value and has fewer calories than meat, as it has less fat. Even oily fish like sardines or anchovies have a smaller quantity of fat (6-8g out of 100g) than those meats which are considered low in fat (chicken 10g out of 100g). The fat in fish has the advantage of not raising the cholesterol level in the blood, although some people find it difficult to digest. Oily fish can be eaten using cooking methods which do not increase their calorific value, such as grilling, baking, pickling etc. White fish have very little fat and can therefore be used in more sophisticated ways, provided that not too many high calorie ingredients are used. This majority of the following fish recipes contain fewer than 200 calories in contrast to the meat recipes, all of which exceed this figure. In addition, fish provides important vitamins and minerals.

PRAWN COCKTAIL

1 lettuce
20 prawns
200g anglerfish
2 sticks celery
100g apple
1 bayleaf
thyme
salt

Sauce:
¼ litre milk
¼ litre olive oil
2 tablespoons ketchup
1 tablespoon brandy
salt
1 lemon

Shred the lettuce into thin strips.
Cook the prawns in salted water and then peel.
Poach the anglerfish in a little salted water with the bayleaf; when cooked, chop into pieces.
Wash the celery and cut into small pieces.
Peel the apples and slice finely; sprinkle the slices with lemon juice.
Take four dishes and at the bottom of each one place a little lettuce, then a tablespoon of the sauce. Pile the rest of the ingredients on top.

To make the sauce: put the oil and milk into a blender and mix until it reaches the consistency of thick mayonnaise. Season with ketchup, brandy, lemon juice and salt.

	Cal.	Pro.	Fat	Carbo.
Per Serving	79	12.9	0.8	3.9
Sauce Total	2.450	8	260	1.8
1 Tbsp	50	0.1	5.2	-

RED MULLET WITH ANCHOVIES

Serves 4

2-3 pieces red mullet per person
4 anchovies
4 tomatoes
8 olives
3 tablespoons fresh parsley
salt
1 lemon
olive oil

Clean the red mullet, season with salt and lemon, brush with the oil, place in an ovenproof dish and cook in a moderate oven for about 20 minutes. Scald the tomatoes, then peel, remove the pips and chop into small pieces.
Sauté the tomatoes for a few minutes in a frying pan with a tablespoon of olive oil, then add the washed and chopped anchovies, the pitted, halved olives and the chopped parsley. Stir for a while, then pour over the fish and serve.

	Cal.	Pro.	Fat	Carbo.
Per Serving	235	37	7.8	4.3

ANGLERFISH IN VINAIGRETTE

Serves 4

800g anglerfish
1 onion, halved
1 bayleaf
50g capers
50g gherkins
3 tomatoes
1 hard-boiled egg

1 tablespoon vinegar
3 tablespoons olive oil
salt and pepper

Cook the fish in a little water with the bayleaf and half the onion, then chop into medium-sized pieces.
Chop the remaining half of the onion as small as possible and make a vinaigrette with a little of the chopped onion, the capers, the gherkins, the boiled egg and the seeded and peeled tomato, finely chopped. Season with salt and pepper, add the oil and vinegar and a few spoonfuls of the fish stock obtained during cooking.
Mix the vinaigrette with the fish and leave to marinate for a couple of hours before eating.

	Cal.	Pro.	Fat	Carbo.
Per Serving	315	34	9.8	6

WHITING WITH GHERKINS

Serves 4

4 whiting
¼ litre white wine
1 onion
4 gherkins
1 dl milk
1 tablespoon cornflour
lemon
½ tablespoon chopped thyme
2 tablespoons chopped parsley

Chop the onion and cook in half a litre of water for about 10 minutes. Add the white wine, thyme and chopped parsley, then place the cleaned whiting into the liquid ensuring that the fish are completely covered. Cook for about 15-20 minutes.
Lift out the fish and place on a plate; add the chopped gherkins to the cooking liquid and thicken with the cornflour dissolved in milk. Season this sauce with salt and lemon and pour over the whiting.

	Cal.	Pro.	Fat	Carbo.
Per Serving	175	34	9.8	6

Top: Anglerfish in Vinaigrette
Bottom: Whiting with Gherkins

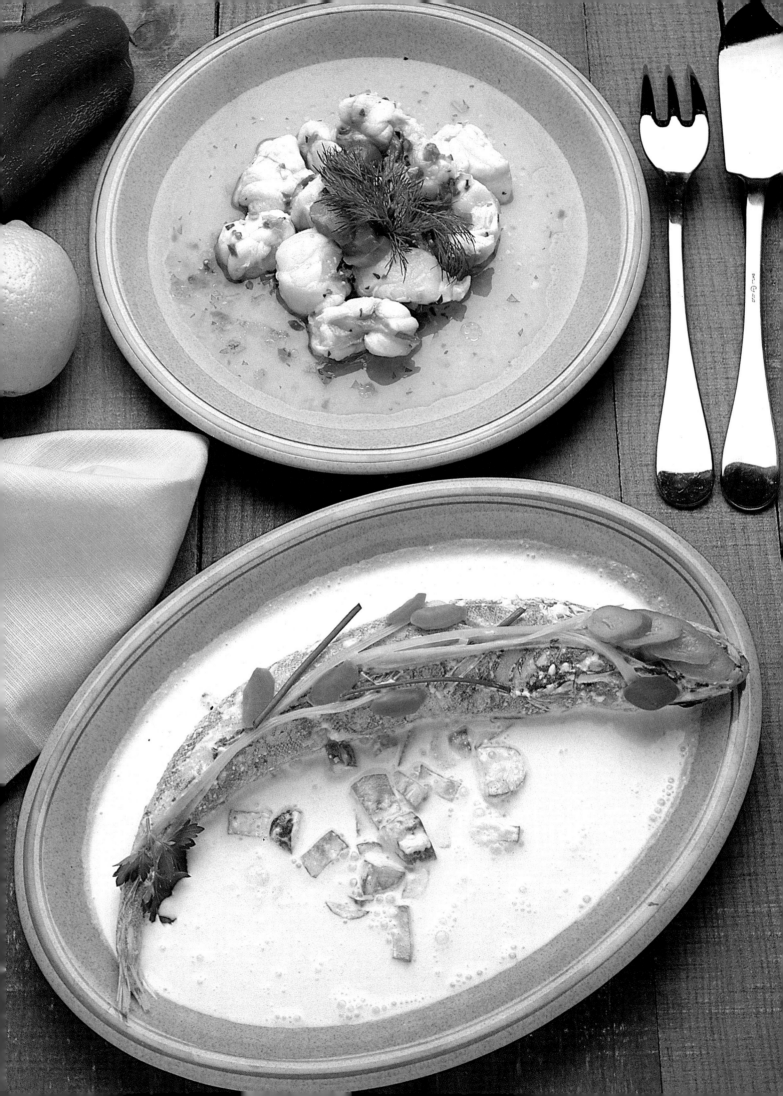

FILLETS OF SOLE WITH MUSSELS

Serves 4

2 large pieces of sole, filleted
1/4 litre white wine
10 mussels
1 leek
1 dl cream
1 bay leaf
pepper and salt

Open the mussels by cooking them with a little white wine, water, salt and a bay leaf.

Remove the mussels and put to one side, and reserve the stock.

Add the stock to the rest of the water and the wine with the chopped leek and some pepper. Simmer for about 20 minutes and strain.

In an ovenproof dish cook the sole fillets with a little of the stock; cook gently so that they do not boil or overcook.

Reduce the rest of the fish stock and add the cream to it. Place the mussels next to the sole fillets and cover with the sauce.

	Cal.	Pro.	Fat	Carbo.
Per Serving	196	25.6	6.7	1.1

COD WITH PEPPERS

Serves 4

400g cod
1/4 litre tomato juice
4 red peppers
1 onion
1 bay leaf
1 tablespoon chopped parsley

Chop the cod into medium sized pieces, cover with cold water and add the bay leaf and the onion chopped into strips. Cook gently for 5 minutes. Drain, then skin the

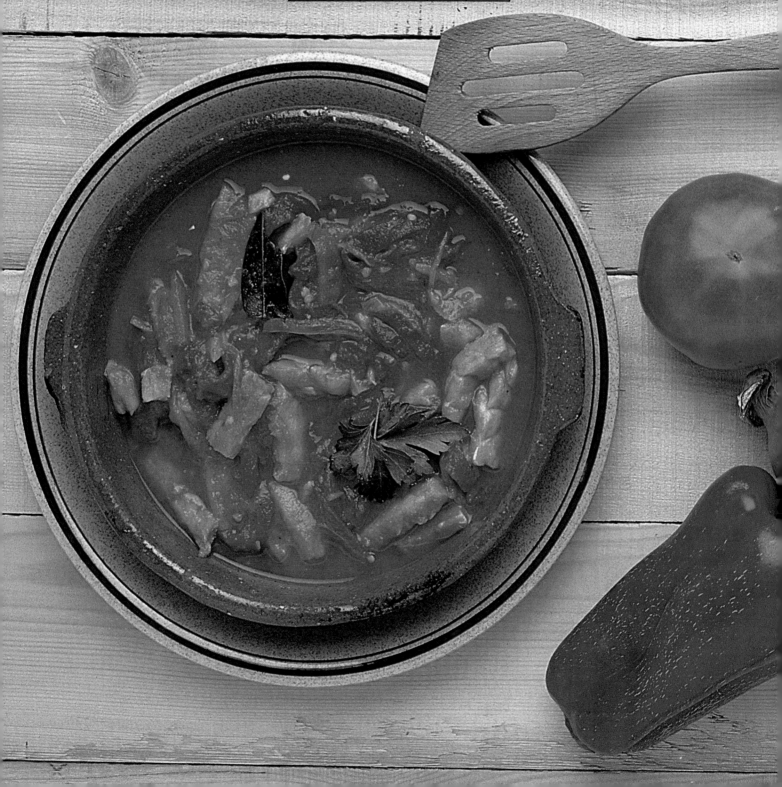

fish and remove the bones.

Roast the peppers in the oven, peel and cut into strips.

In an ovenproof dish, greased with olive oil, pour some tomato sauce, then make a layer of pepper strips, then pieces of cod, then cover with more tomatoes and peppers etc.

Cook for a few minutes in the oven and serve sprinkled with parsley.

	Cal.	Pro.	Fat	Carbo.
Per Serving	140	17.7	5.6	5.3

STUFFED TROUT

Serves 4

4 trout
½ onion
1 clove garlic
1 dessertspoon paprika
1 tablespoon chopped parsley
2 tablespoons vinegar
3 slices toast
2 tablspoons olive oil
1 lemon

Clean and fillet the trout, season with salt and a little lemon juice.

Mix together the crushed garlic, paprika, parsley, crumbled toast and salt. Add to it the oil and vinegar and the finely chopped onion and blend well (all of this could be done in a liquidizer).

Divide the stuffing between the trout. Wrap up each one separately in aluminium foil and roast in a low oven for about 15 minutes. Serve wrapped in the foil.

	Cal.	Pro.	Fat	Carbo.
Per Serving	177	20.5	7.3	7.2

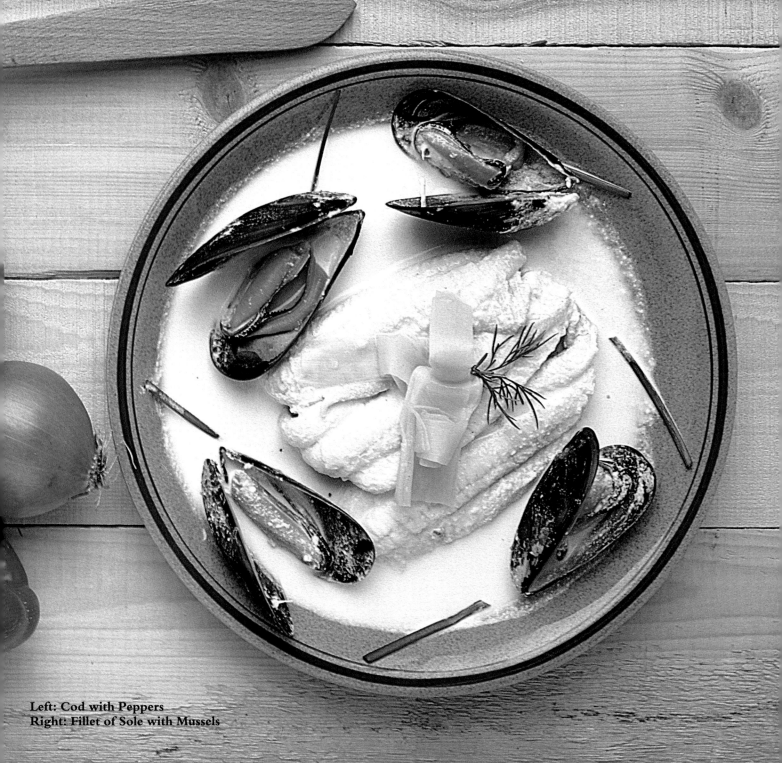

Left: Cod with Peppers
Right: Fillet of Sole with Mussels

DORADE WITH COCKLES

Serves 4

1 dorade
2 large onions
20 cockles
1/4 litre cider
1 teaspoon paprika
1 bay leaf
2 tablespoons olive oil
chopped parsley
salt

Put the cleaned dorade in an ovenproof dish and cover with water. Add the chopped onions, cider, paprika, olive oil and salt. Cook on a low heat for 30 minutes. Put the cockles in a saucepan with a little salted water and a bay leaf. Take them off the heat when they open. Drain and keep the stock.

Remove the fish from the oven. Add to the fish stock the stock from the cockles and put the mixture in a blender. Cover the fish with this sauce and garnish with the cockles. Heat in the oven for a few minutes and serve with chopped parsley.

This recipe can be made using hake, anglerfish or eel.

	Cal.	Pro.	Fat	Carbo.
Per Serving	209	24	8.6	9

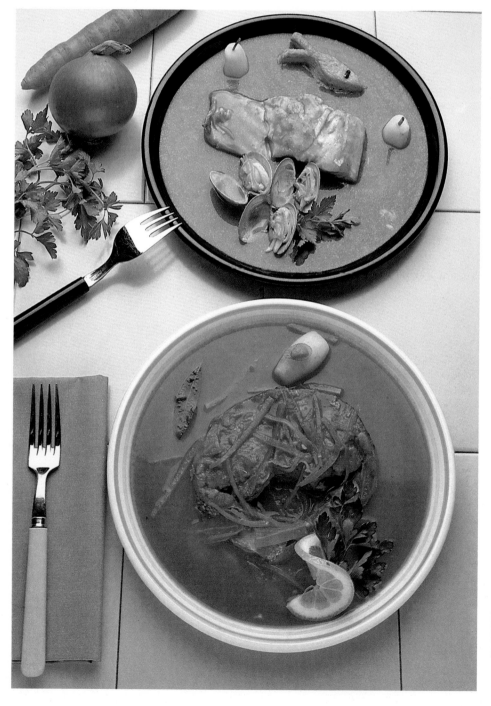

HAKE IN BRANDY

Serves 4

4 x 200g hake fillets
300g carrots
250g onions
1 dl tomato juice
1 bay leaf
1 dl brandy
juice of 1/2 lemon
salt

Chop the carrots and onions finely and cook in a pan in about a glassful of water (they can also be cooked in a pressure cooker) until soft, adding more water if necessary although the mixture should not become soup-like.

Add the brandy, bay leaf and tomato juice, and when it boils, add the hake seasoned with salt and the lemon juice. Cook for about 20 minutes.

When the fish is cooked, transfer to the serving dish and pour the sauce on top.

	Cal.	Pro.	Fat	Carbo.
Per Serving	200	33.6	1.6	13

SOUSED TROUT IN RED WINE

Serves 4

4 trout
2 litres water
1/4 litre red wine
1/4 litre vinegar
2 carrots
2 onions
salt
black peppercorns
lemon
bay leaf
parsley

Clean the trout and soak in boiling vinegar for at least 30 minutes. Meanwhile add the red wine to the water, then the chopped onion and carrot, the bay leaf and a few black peppercorns. Cook this mixture for 15 minutes then add the trout and cook gently for a further 10-15 minutes. The trout can be served hot or cold, seasoned with salt and garnished with chopped parsley and lemon slices.

	Cal.	Pro.	Fat	Carbo.
Per Serving	181	32	2.2	19

Dorade with Cockles (top)
Hake in Brandy   (bottom)

MEAT DISHES

Meat provides our diet with valuable proteins as well as important vitamins and minerals such as iron. The calorie content of meat is proportional to its fat content. The meats lowest in fat are chicken and veal.

It is advisable to roast or grill meat or to make simple stews with few fatty ingredients. Here are some recipes to add variety to the diet.

VEAL FILLETS NEAPOLITAN

Serves 4

4 x 100g veal fillets
4 x 50g slices of cheese
4 tomatoes
3 teaspoons fresh or 2 teaspoons dried oregano
salt
sugar
olive oil

Prepare the fillets by removing any fat. Cook them in a non-stick frying pan. Place the fillets in an ovenproof dish and on each one place a thin slice of tomato and a slice of cheese, then sprinkle with oregano and salt.

Put into the oven for a few minutes until the cheese melts, but do not let the meat dry out.

Roast the remaining tomatoes in the oven - cut in half and sprinkle with oregano, parsley and a little sugar . When cooked, season and drizzle a little olive oil over them. Serve with the fillets.

	Cal.	Pro.	Fat	Carbo.
Per Serving	*304*	*22.1*	*2.2*	*6.5*

CHICKEN WITH FRUIT

Serves 4

1 chicken
4 slices of pineapple
2 apples
1 dl white wine
1 tablespoon grated coconut
approx. 1 teaspoon curry powder
stock

salt & pepper
juice of ¹/₂ lemon
olive oil

Chop the chicken into large pieces and season with salt, pepper and lemon juice. In a casserole dish with a lid brown the chicken pieces in a little olive oil over a gentle heat, until the juices run from the chicken and it is golden brown. Then drain off the fat, leaving just the chicken in the dish.

Add the white wine and let it cook for 15 minutes. Add the grated coconut, apple and pineapple slices. Season with curry

	Cal.	Pro.	Fat	Carbo.
Per Serving	*290*	*20*	*11.6*	*27*

Top: Veal Fillets Neapolitan
Bottom: Chicken with Fruit

powder to taste and cook until the apple is soft. If desired, it can be thickened with cornflour dissolved in cold water (1 tablespoon is approximately 35 calories).

FILLET STEAK WITH TOMATO

Serves 4

4 x 100g fillet steaks
2 large onions, cut into rings
400g mushrooms
2 dl tomato juice
pepper and salt
olive oil

Prepare the steaks by beating them and cutting off any fat or sinewy parts. Cook in a non-stick frying pan with a small amount of oil. Put the onion rings into an oven-proof dish and place the steaks on top. Add the mushrooms (whole), the tomato juice and a little stock. Cook for a

Below, top: Fillet Steak with Tomato
Below, bottom: Veal and Anchovy Roll
Opposite, top: Chicken with Olives and Carrots (recipe on page 48)
Opposite, bottom: Chicken in Beer

few minutes, then check to see if the meat is tender and the sauce cooked. Let the sauce reduce a little by cooking with the lid off.

Serve the steaks covered in the sauce and mushrooms.

	Cal.	Pro.	Fat	Carbo.
Per Serving	*258*	*21*	*17*	*5*

VEAL AND ANCHOVY ROLL

Serves 6

500g finely minced veal
3 eggs
10 anchovies
1 dl dry sherry
salt and pepper

Wash the anchovies to remove the oil from the tin, chop them and add them, to the veal. Then mix with the sherry, beaten eggs and pepper. Season, taking care not to add too much salt as the anchovies are already very salty. Fill a long mould or loaf tin with the meat mixture and cook in the oven for 45 minutes.

Unmould and cut when cold. Serve with a salad.

	Cal.	Pro.	Fat	Carbo.
Per Serving	*249*	*20*	*18*	*0.1*

CHICKEN IN BEER

Serves 4

1 chicken
2 large onions, chopped into rings
1 clove garlic, crushed
1 small bottle of beer
salt & pepper
juice of 1/2 lemon

Quarter the chicken. Put the onion rings in an ovenproof casserole dish, and on top place the chicken seasoned with salt, pepper, lemon juice and garlic. Put into a moderate oven and cook until golden, taking care that the onions do not burn. Then cover with the beer. Cover and cook for about 15 minutes (the beer loses its calories as the alcohol evaporates during cooking). Serve with the onions, which can be liquidized if desired.

	Cal.	Pro.	Fat	Carbo.
Per Serving	*200*	*21*	*11*	*10*

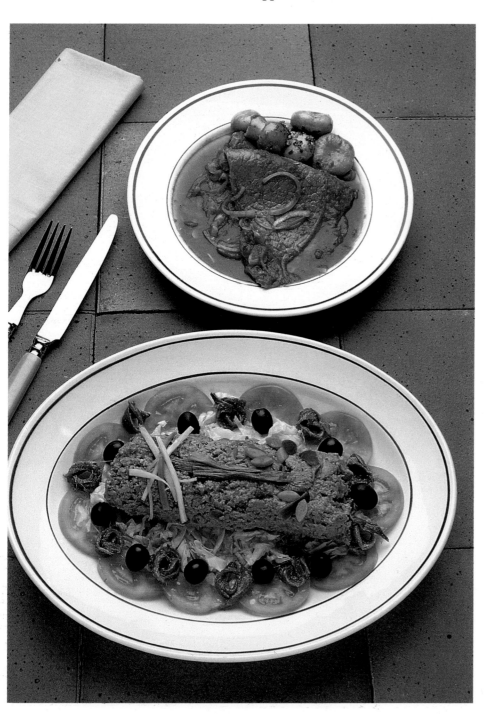

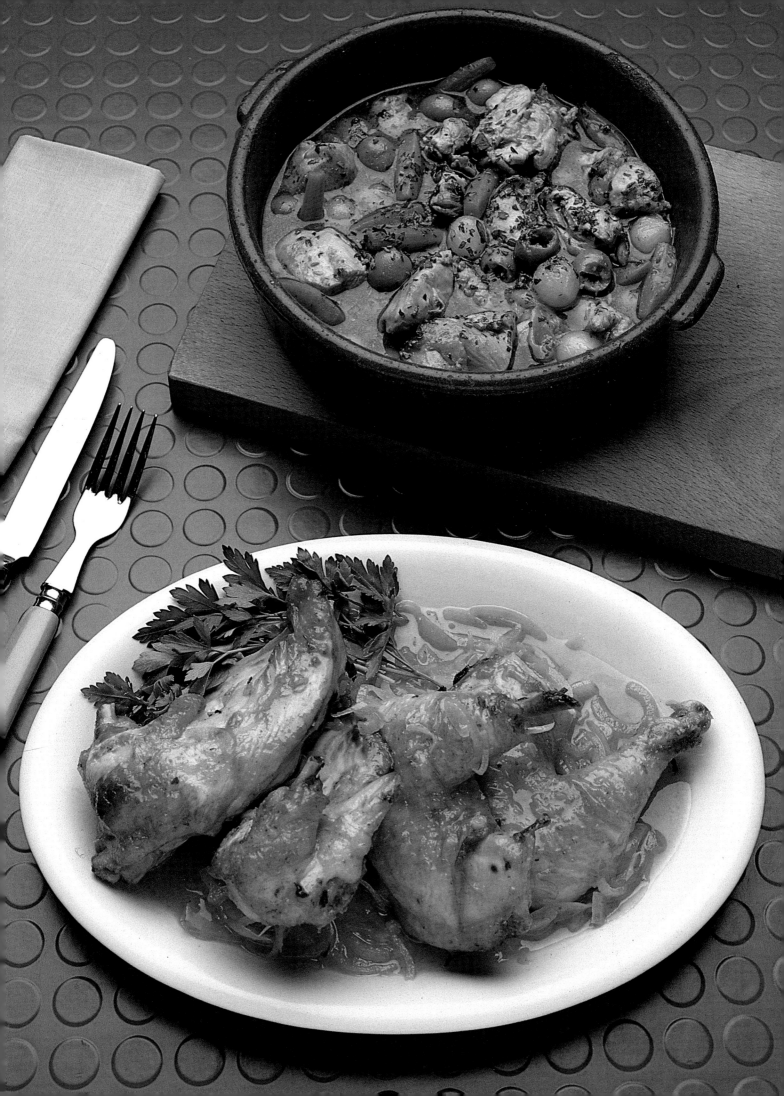

MEAT KEBABS

4 chicken breasts or 400g chopped veal
4 cherry tomatoes
2 roast peppers
4 fresh or tinned artichokes
½ glass brandy
juice of 1 lemon
salt & pepper
2 cloves garlic, crushed
olive oil

Chop the chicken breasts into bite-sized pieces and marinate in a mixture of the lemon juice , brandy and crushed garlic, seasoned with salt and pepper.

Alternate the meat, pepper slices, artichokes and tomatoes on skewers. If

Left: Meat Kebabs
Right: Hamburgers with peppers

the tomatoes are large they can be roasted as an accompaniment. Barbecue, roast in the oven, or grill, using just a little oil to baste.

	Cal.	Pro.	Fat	Carbo.
Per Serving	240	21.8	13.4	7.6

CHICKEN WITH OLIVES AND CARROTS

Serves 4

300g pickling onions
300g carrots
24 pitted green olives
a little white wine
salt & pepper
1 tablespoon chopped parsley
olive oil

Chop the chicken and season with salt and pepper; fry it in hot olive oil (the chicken loses its own fat during frying and although it absorbs a little oil, the final result is not high in calories). Drain well.

Cook the pickling onions and finely sliced carrots in salted water.

Place the chicken in a pan. Add the cooked onions and carrots and the olives. Add the white wine and allow to reduce

(the alcohol loses its calorific value during cooking).

When reduced add a little of the stock from the vegetables and cook for a few minutes.

Serve in an earthenware dish, sprinkled with parsley.

	Cal.	Pro.	Fat	Carbo.
Per Serving	280	22	12.7	14

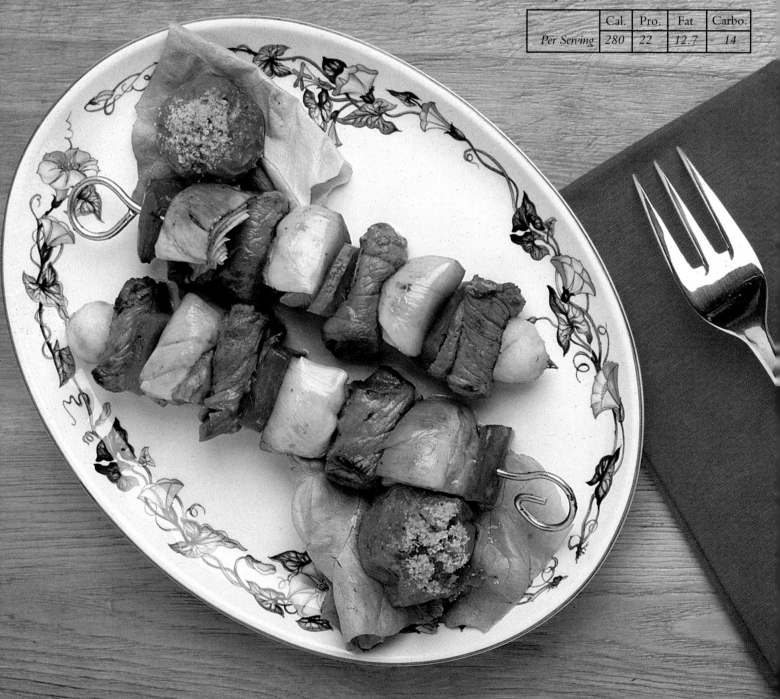

HAMBURGERS WITH PEPPERS

500g minced veal
1 egg
1 onion
1 dl milk
500g red peppers
2 cloves garlic, crushed
1 tablespoon olive oil
salt and pepper

Chop the onion and cook in a little water. Drain carefully so it is almost dry, and add the milk.

Beat the egg into the meat, add the onion and milk and season with salt and pepper.

Make the hamburgers and cook in a non-stick frying pan.

Serve with roast peppers – roast the peppers dry in the oven; when roasted peel and cut into strips. Brown the crushed garlic in the oil and sauté the peppers.

	Cal.	Pro.	Fat	Carbo.
Per Serving	352	28.8	25	9

BEEF STEW WITH RICE

Serves 4

500g chopped stewing steak
2 large onions
2 cloves garlic, crushed
1 tablespoon paprika
100g rice
1 dl tomato juice
olive oil
1 bayleaf
¾ litre stock

Remove the fat from the meat, season and brown in a little oil with the garlic. When golden, drain off all the oil, leaving only the meat. Sprinkle with the paprika, stirring continuously to prevent it from burning, then cover with stock. Add the finely chopped onion and tomato juice. Season with the bayleaf, salt and pepper and cook until the meat is tender (about 1 hour). If necessary, add more stock.

Serve with white rice which has been boiled in plenty of water.

	Cal.	Pro.	Fat	Carbo.
Per Serving	340	19	17	23

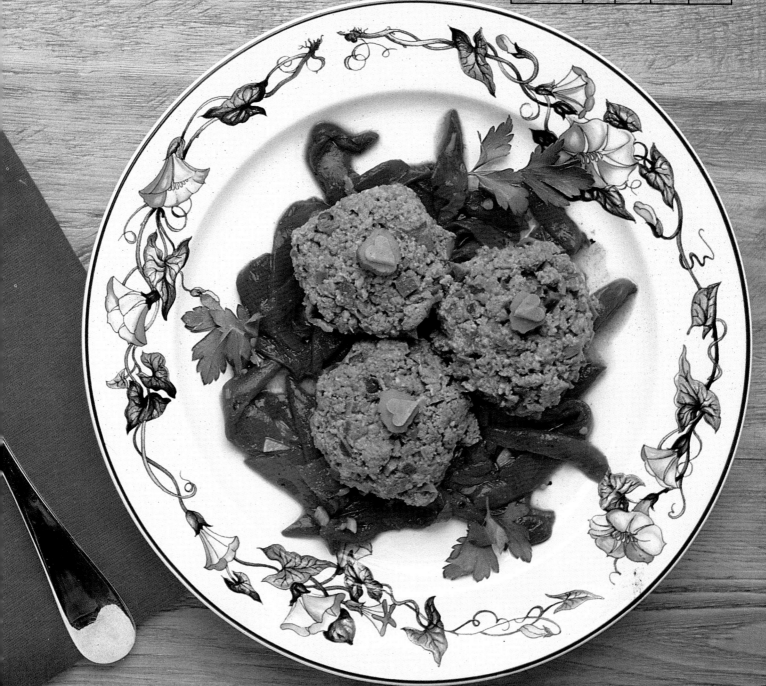

LIGHT LUNCH AND SUPPER DISHES

Cheese, cold meats and even pancakes and pies - in the correct proportions - can constitute dishes with an acceptable level of calories, depending on the number of calories allowed in the diet.

MINI HAM ROLLS

Serves 4

4 x 70g slices of York ham
1 x 75g banana
3 large (400g) apples
juice of 1 lemon
50g Cheddar cheese
50g cornflakes

Grate the apples and coat with lemon juice. Add to this the mashed banana, cubed cheese and crushed cornflakes. Spreak the mixture on the ham slices and roll up.

	Cal.	Pro.	Fat	Carbo.
Per Serving	320	17.4	15.5	27.5

PARMA HAM WITH FRESH TOMATO SAUCE

Serves 4

4 x 70g slices Parma ham
400g tomatoes
100g pitted olives
25g capers
1 hard-boiled egg
8 asparagus spears, cooked
2 tablespoons olive oil
oregano
salt

Remove any fat from the parma ham. Make a sauce with the scalded, peeled and diced tomato, the olives, capers and the chopped hard-boiled egg. Drizzle over some olive oil and season with oregano and salt.

Serve the ham with the asparagus and the tomato sauce on the side.

	Cal.	Pro.	Fat	Carbo.
Per Serving	390	14.5	33	8

FOLDED CREPES

Serves 4

2 eggs
1 dl milk
1 large tomato
2 x 100g slices York ham
100g Cheddar cheese
olive oil (to grease pan)
tarragon
salt

Beat the eggs with the milk. Season, and in a non-stick pan, make four thin pancakes, cooking until golden on both sides.

Inside each one, put a slice of tomato and a little bit of cheese, then fold over the edge taking care the filling does not come out.

	Cal.	Pro.	Fat	Carbo.
Per Serving	235	16.2	16.8	3.2

YORK HAM WITH ASPARAGUS

Serves 4

4 x 100g slices York Ham
200g frozen mixed vegetables (carrots, peas, beans, etc.)
12 asparagus spears
2 tbsp mayonnaise
4 tbsp yogurt

Cook the mixed vegetables in salted water. Drain and allow to cool. Mix the mayonnaise with the yogurt and spread this mixture thinly onto each slice of ham, mixing the rest with the salad. Place the salad on the ham slices; place an asparagus spear in the middle and roll the ham, so that the asparagus tips emerge from either end of the roll.

	Cal.	Pro.	Fat	Carbo.
Per Serving	328	21.6	23.3	8

SALAD CREPES

Serves 4

2 eggs
1 dl milk
200g lettuce
4 anchovies
1 tin artichoke hearts
1 small tin asparagus tips
2 tablespoons olive oil
1 tablespoon vinegar
pepper and salt

Beat the eggs with the milk, season with salt and pepper and make four thin pancakes in a non-stick omelette pan.

Wash the lettuce and chop into thin strips. Cut the artichokes into quarters. Wash the anchovies and chop into small pieces. Mix together the lettuce, artichokes, asparagus and anchovies. Dress with the olive oil and vinegar, fill the pancakes with this mixture and fold them in half.

	Cal.	Pro.	Fat	Carbo.
Per Serving	140	7	9.3	6.1

**Top: York Ham with Asparagus
Bottom: Rice Medley (recipe on page 56)**

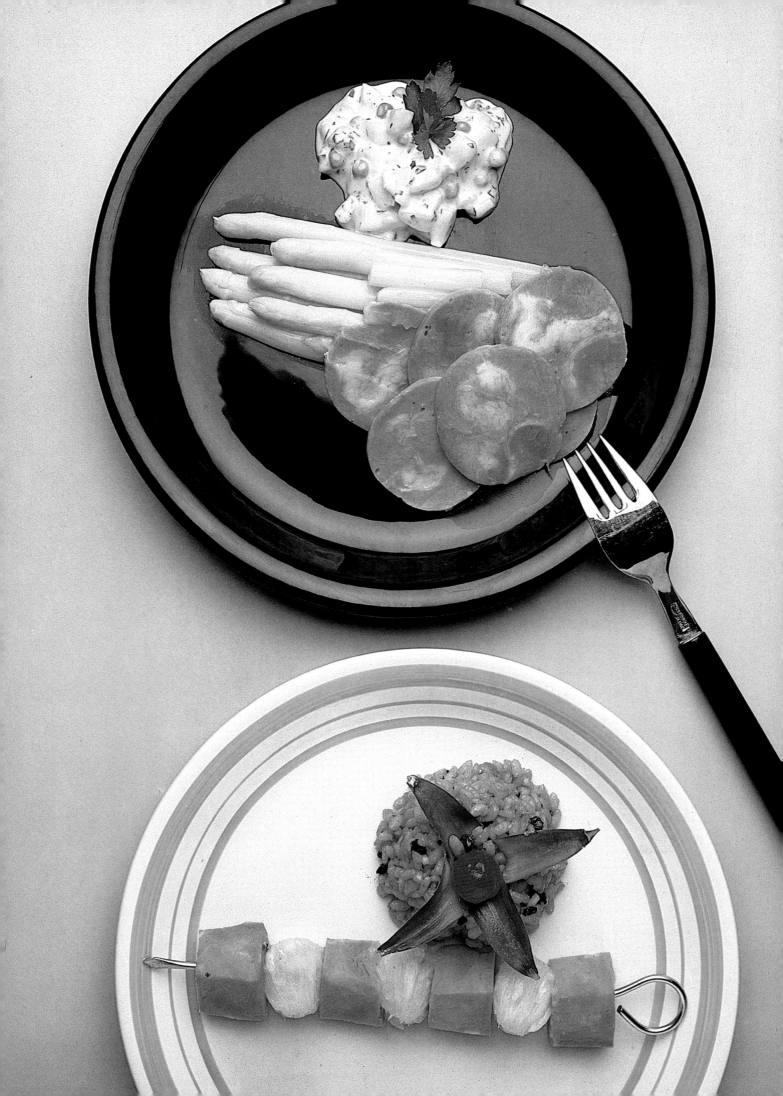

YORK HAM WITH PINEAPPLE

Serves 4

4 x 70g slices York ham
1 tin (8 slices) pineapple
1 tablespoon (10g) sugar
10g butter

Melt the butter in a frying pan, and sauté the York ham, then place the ham in a dish. Add the sugar to the melted butter, stirring well until it caramelises. Add 2 dl of the syrup from the pineapples and half the chopped pineapple. Cook for a few minutes and then cover the ham with this mixture.

Decorate with the remaining pineapple slices.

	Cal.	Pro.	Fat	Carbo.
Per Serving	*440*	*13.9*	*37*	*12*

CHEESE TOASTIE

Serves 4

4 x 100g slices cheese
4 thin slices bread
100g mushrooms
100g carrots
100g apple
juice of 1/2 lemon
salt and pepper

Slice the mushrooms and sprinkle with the lemon juice. Season with salt and pepper. Grate the carrot and apple and add to the mushroom mixture.

Toast the sliced bread; on top of each piece of toast place a slice of cheese and then divide the mushroom mixture into four potions and spread on top of the cheese on each slice.

	Cal.	Pro.	Fat	Carbo.
Per Serving	*214*	*11.7*	*8*	*23.8*

Cheese Toastie

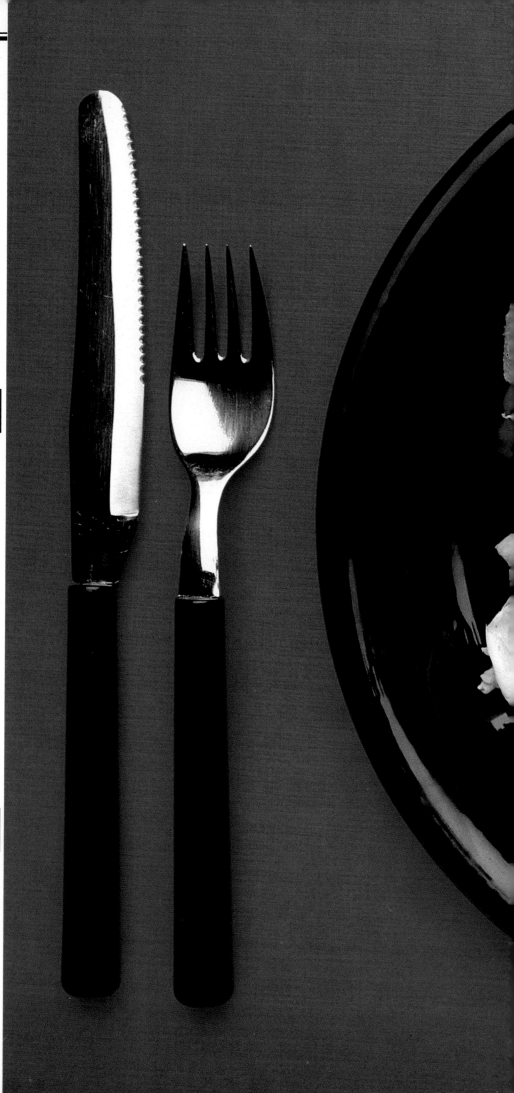

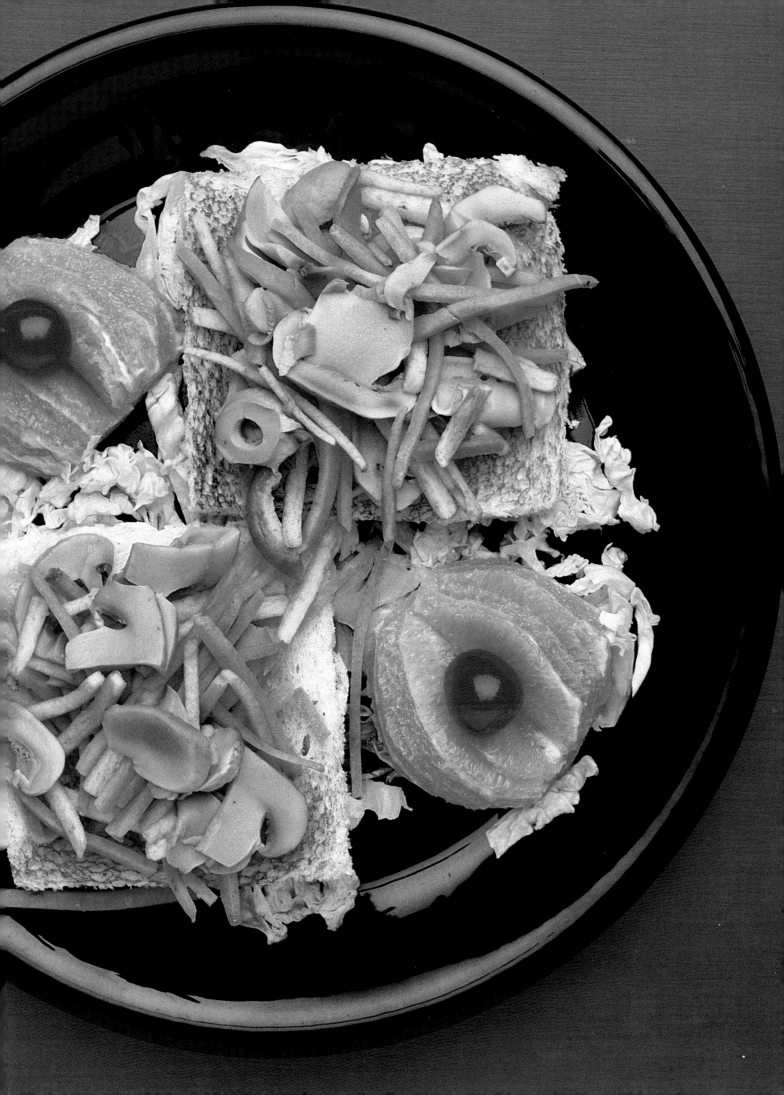

FISH PIE

Serves 4

Pastry:
200g flour
½ glass water
40g yeast
salt

Filling:
500g hake fillets or steaks
2 tablespoons olive oil
saffron
pepper and salt

To make the pastry, dissolve the yeast in tepid water and mix in the flour a little at a time – it may not all be needed – until a soft dough is produced. Knead it a little until it is elastic and let it stand for 30 minutes until it's doubled in volume.

Crush a few saffron seeds in a mortar (dish) with a little salt. When it is powdery, mix with pepper and the olive oil and marinate the fish in this mixture. Roll out the pastry quite thinly with a rolling pin and cut out eight circles, 12cm in diameter. Place a little of the fish

mixture in the centre of four of the circles, then cover with the four remaining pastry circles. Press the edges together with water, and glaze with a beaten egg. Cook in a moderate oven for about 30 minutes.

	Cal.	Pro.	Fat	Carbo.
Per Serving	*317*	*26*	*6.3*	*37.5*

ARGENTINIAN PIES

Serves 4

Pastry:
200g flour
½ glass water
30g yeast
salt

Filling:
100g onion
200g potatoes
300g minced veal
3 tablespoons concentrated stock
1 egg
pepper & salt

To make the pastry, dissolve the yeast in tepid water, add the salt and flour, mixing until a soft dough is formed (depending on the type of flour, not all of the 200g may be required, so add it a little at a time). Allow to rise in a warm place until it doubles in volume.

Filling: Finely chop the onion and mix with the minced meat, the beaten egg, the stock and the finely diced potato. Season with salt and pepper.

Roll out the pastry thinly and cut eight circles, 12cm in diameter. Divide the filling between four of the circles and cover with the remaining four. Press the edges together well and glaze the pastry with beaten egg. Cook in a low oven for approximately 1 hour.

	Cal.	Pro.	Fat	Carbo.
Per Serving	*370*	*18*	*10.4*	*49.4*

Fish Pies

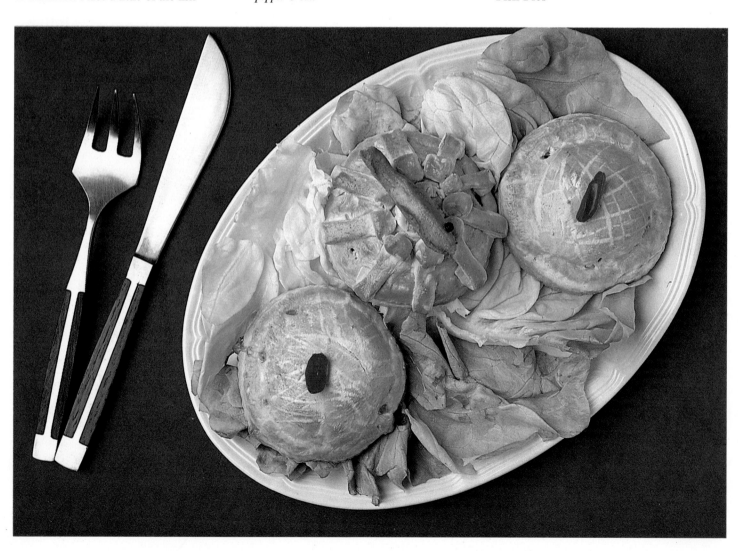

SNACKS

It is becoming increasingly common to replace complete meals with light snacks and easily prepared dishes.

Because these snacks are usually a substitute for proper meals, they should contain a balanced list of ingredients: protein, from meat, fish, eggs or cheese, some kind of vegetable, and a carbohydrate element, such as rice, potatoes, bread. Ingredients which are high in energy, such as dried fruits, can also be used sparingly.

CHEESE SNACK

Serves 4

4 x 100g slices of cheese
4 thin slices tomato
2 bananas
4 slices bread
200g lettuce
2 large oranges
3 tablespoons olive oil
salt

On each slice of bread place a slice of tomato, a cheese slice and half a sliced banana. Put into a low oven for ten minutes. Peel the orange and separate into segments, then wash and chop the lettuce. Mix the lettuce and orange segments together and dress with the olive oil and salt. Serve as an accompaniment to the cheese toasts.

	Cal.	Pro.	Fat	Carbo.
Per Serving	354	13	15	39.4

COLD PLATTER

Serves 4

4 eggs
12 spears asparagus
2 x 100g slices York ham
1 small tin artichokes

For the sauce:
1 dl milk
1 dl olive oil
1 tablespoon mustard
Salt

Hard-boil the eggs for 12 minutes, then peel. Cut each slice of ham in half lengthways. If the tinned artichokes are very acidic, cook for a few minutes in boiling water and drain.

Sauce: Put the ingredients in a liquidizer and blend to the consistency of a thick mayonnaise.

Top: Parma Ham with Fresh Tomato Sauce (recipe on page 50)
Bottom: Cheese snack

On four plates put a boiled egg in the middle, 3 asparagus spears rolled inside half a slice of ham, three or four artichokes and a spoonful of sauce.

	Cal.	Pro.	Fat	Carbo.
Per Serving	82	5.1	4	3.7
Sauce Total	965	3.3	104	0.9
1 Tbsp	53	0.1	5.7	-

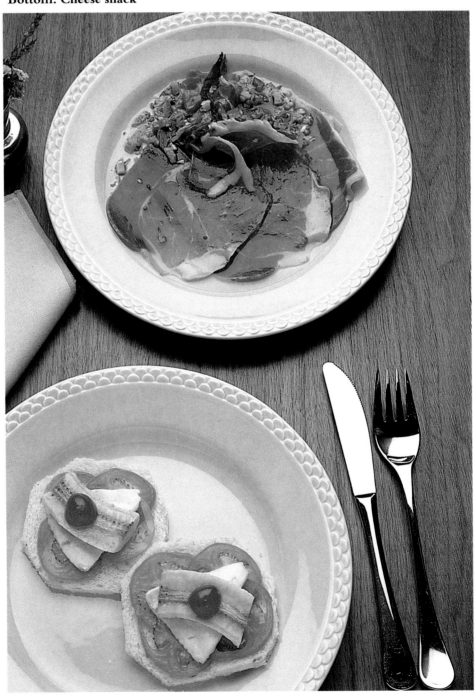

CHICKEN SNACK

Serves 4

4 chicken breasts
2 slices pineapple
2 apples
80g rice
150g cheese
juice of 1 lemon
20g butter
1 tablespoon chopped parsley

Cook the rice in plenty of water, then drain. Cut the apples into quarters, then cook in a little water and lemon juice. Grill the chicken breasts.

Put the chicken breasts on to four plates and arrange on each one 2 slices of cooked apple, half a pineapple slice and diced cheese mixed with the rice.

In a small frying pan melt the butter and when hot add the chopped parsley and juice of a lemon. Spoon this mixture onto the rice on each plate.

	Cal.	Pro.	Fat	Carbo.
Per Serving	332	23.4	17	18.9

RICE MEDLEY

Serves 4

120g rice
4 chopped slices pineapple

400g York ham pieces
4 medium apples
1 banana
500g raisins
3 tablespoons sunflower oil
1 tablespoon sugar

Take 4 skewers and thread on the ham pieces alternating with the pineapple chunks. Put the oil into a frying pan and brown the kebabs. Then sauté the diced banana, apple and raisins. Add the sugar and a few spoonfuls of water so the apples cook, and leave for a few minutes until the fruit softens and absorbs the water. Cook the rice in plenty of salted water. Drain and mix with the fruit. Serve this mixture to accompany each kebab.

	Cal.	Pro.	Fat	Carbo.
Per Serving	560	22	28	53

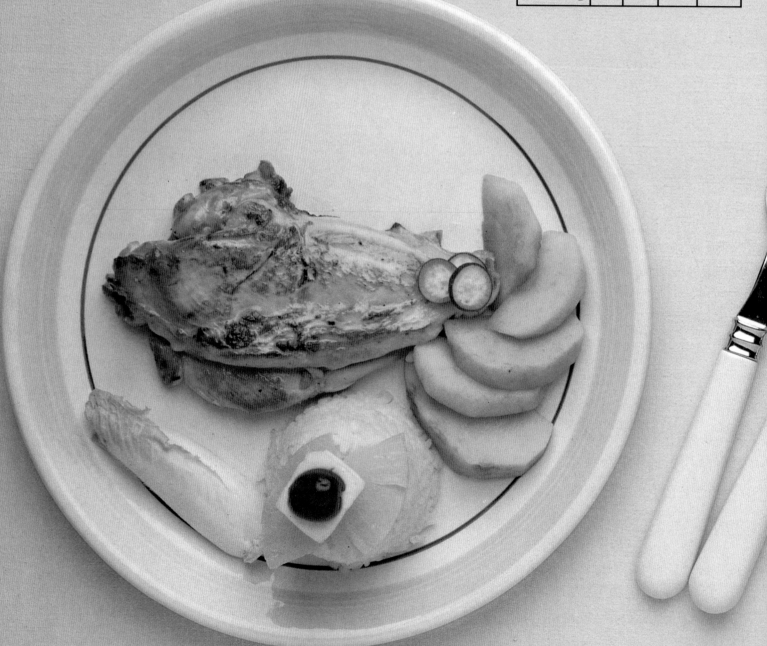

PARMA HAM SURPRISE

Serves 4

4 x 100g slices Parma ham
¼ litre tomato juice
1 lb cooked and mashed potato
500g green beans

Cook the slices of parma ham in a non-stick frying pan. Cook the fresh or frozen green beans in salted water. Drain. Divide the ham slices between four plates, then add the mashed potatoes and the green beans. Serve with hot tomato sauce.

	Cal.	Pro.	Fat	Carbo.
Per Serving	490	19.5	31.4	32

POTATOES WITH EGGS

Serves 4

4 x 100g potatoes
4 eggs
4 small tomatoes
8 anchovies
fresh or dried thyme

Wash the potatoes, prick with a fork, and wrap in aluminium foil. Bake in the oven for 1½-2 hours until soft.
  Drain and rinse the anchovies. Wash the tomatoes, cut in half and place an anchovy on top of each half. Sprinkle with thyme. Roast in the oven until very soft.
  Fry the eggs in a non-stick pan.

On each plate serve an egg, the jacket potato still in the foil and 2 portions of roast tomato.

	Cal.	Pro.	Fat	Carbo.
Per Serving	224	14	7.7	23.6

Left: Parma Ham Surprise
Right: Chicken Snack

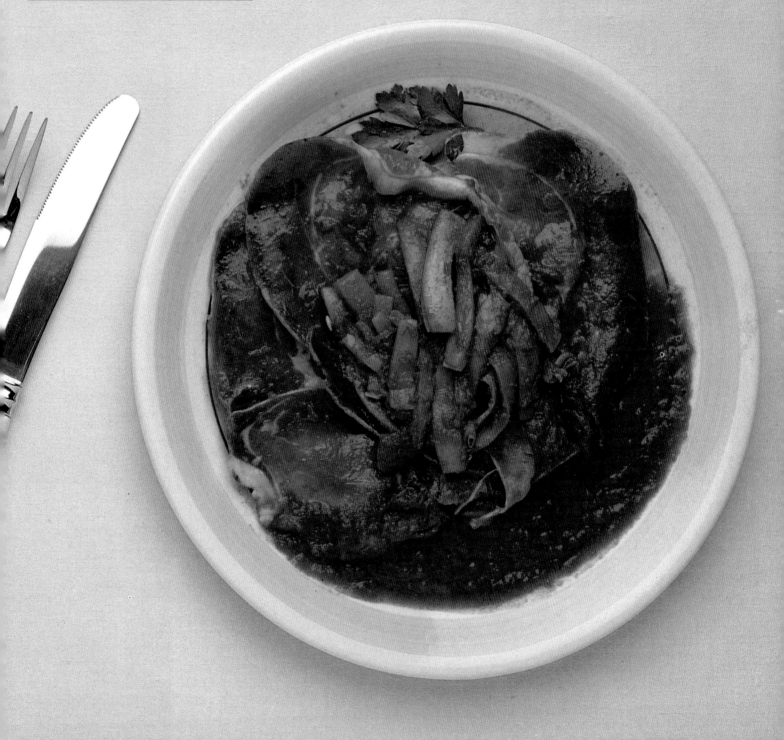

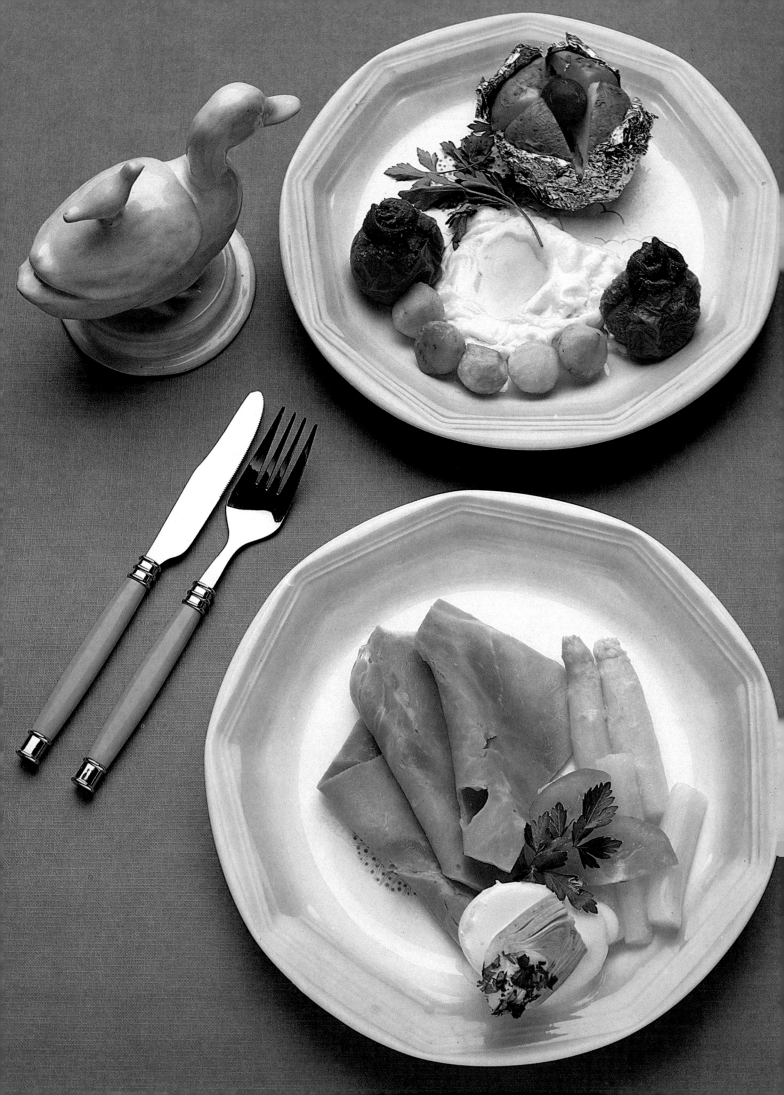

DESSERTS

The most effective dessert for slimmers is always fruit. It is also the healthiest option, as fruit provides a great quantity of vitamins and minerals as well as fibre.

The majority of desserts are highly calorific, but the following – mainly fruit-based recipes – have been carefully selected because of their relatively low calorie count.

LEMON FOAM

Serves 6

6 egg whites
250g sugar
2 dl lemon juice
2 leaves gelatine
1 lemon

Dissolve the gelatine in 2 tablespoons of water and heat gently in a pan.

Beat the egg whites and the sugar into stiff peaks. Then add the warm gelatine mixture a little at a time, constantly beating, followed by the juice and grated rind of the lemon.

Pour into a sundae dish or glass bowl and allow to set in the fridge.

	Cal.	Pro.	Fat	Carbo.
Per Serving	230	5.5	-	46

APRICOT COMPOTE

Serves 4

4 small apricots
2 tablespoons sugar
¼ litre water (approx)
1 dl single cream

Wash the apricots. Put them in a saucepan, cover with the water and add the sugar. Heat, and when the water begins to boil, skim off any scum. Cover and remove

from the heat to allow the fruit to soften.

When lukewarm, carefully remove the apricots and reduce the syrup by cooking it until 1 dl remains. Mix this with the cream and cover the apricots with it.

	Cal.	Pro.	Fat	Carbo.
Per Serving	124	1.2	6	16

STRAWBERRY FOAM

Serves 6

200g strawberries
150g sugar
4 egg whites
2 dl single cream
3 leaves gelatine
juice of 1 lemon

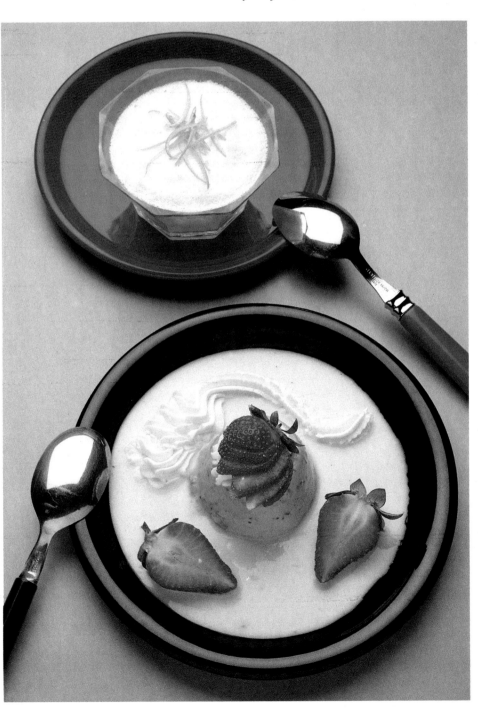

Left, top: Potatoes with Egg (recipe on page 57)
Left, bottom: Cold Platter (recipe on page 55)
Right, top: Lemon Foam
Right, bottom: Strawberry Foam

Wash the strawberries and soak in 50g of sugar and the lemon juice. Chop the strawberries until they resemble a purée. Whip the cream (without sugar) and put aside. Dissolve the gelatine in 2 tablespoons of water, and heat in a pan, stirring constantly. Whip the egg whites with the remaining 100g of sugar and add the gelatine mixture, constantly beating. Add the strawberries then gently fold in the whipped cream. Turn into a mould and cool in the fridge. Unmould and decorate with mint leaves.

	Cal.	Pro.	Fat	Carbo.
Per Serving	220	3.2	8	29

APPLE CREPES

Pancakes:
60g flour
2 eggs
1 dl milk
salt

Filling:
3 apples
rind of 1 orange
2 tablespoons sugar
2 tablespoons brandy

Pancakes: Mix the milk into the flour, stirring well so there are no lumps. Add the eggs and mix well. Season.

Melt a little butter in a non-stick omelette pan and make about 12 thin pancakes.

Filling: Peel and chop the apples and cook them over a gentle heat with the sugar, brandy and orange rind. Mix in a liquidizer or blender to make a smooth purée.

Fill each pancake with a layer of apple purée, fold over and serve hot or cold.

	Cal.	Pro.	Fat	Carbo.
Per Serving	184	5.8	4.2	30.7

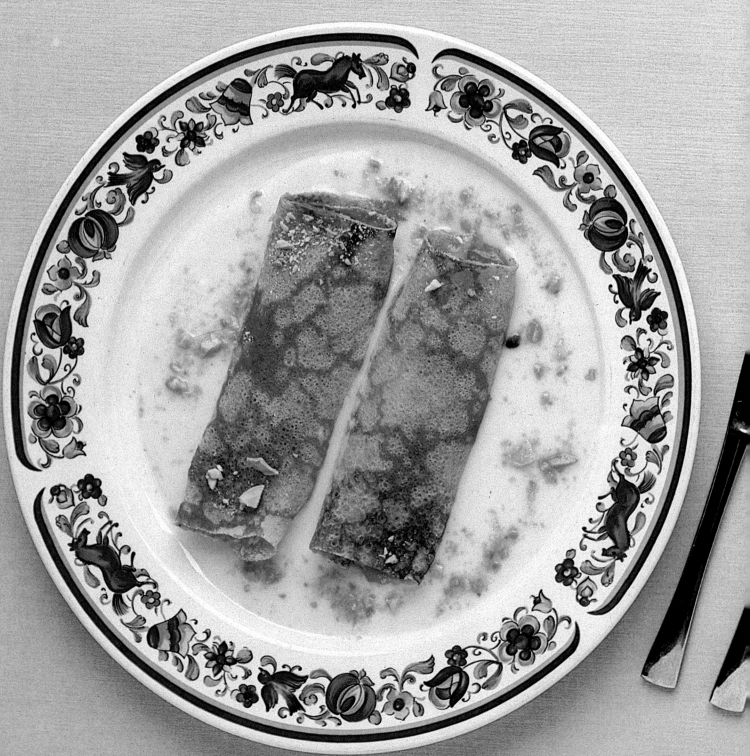

FRUIT KEBABS

Serves 4

1 banana
3 tangerines
12 strawberries
4 slices pineapple
1 small melon
3 tablespoons Kirsch
juice of 1 orange

Slice the banana. Peel the tangerines and
separate into segments. Wash the
strawberries and chop the pineapple. Cube
the melon or use a scoop to make small
melon balls.

Put all of the fruit pieces onto skewers.
Melt a little butter in a pan and add the
sugar and allow to brown for a short
while, then add the Kirsch and orange
juice. Sprinkle this mixture over the
kebabs.

	Cal.	Pro.	Fat	Carbo.
Per Serving	115	1	2.9	21.5

Left: Apple Pancakes
Right: Stuffed Oranges

STUFFED ORANGES

Serves 4

4 large oranges
300g carrots
3 tablespoons sugar
1 small tub of yoghurt

Cut off the top part of the orange so it
forms a lid, hollow out the flesh and blend
it in a liquidizer to make a smooth purée.
Set aside. Cook the carrots in a little water
– while still hot, chop and add to it the
orange flesh with the sugar.

Mix it with the yoghurt and use to fill
the oranges. Serve cold.

	Cal.	Pro.	Fat	Carbo.
Per Serving	125	2.9	1.3	26.4

FRUIT CREPES

Pancakes:
60g flour

2 eggs
1 dl milk
butter
salt

Filling:
200g strawberries
1 banana
1 tablespoon sugar
lemon juice and crystallised sugar

Pancakes: Mix the milk with the flour,
mixing well so no lumps form. Add the
eggs and mix well. Season.

Melt a little butter in a non-stick
omelette pan and make thin pancakes.
Filling: Wash and slice the strawberries,
cut the banana into small pieces and cover
with the lemon juice and sugar. Fill each
pancake with the fruit mixture and
sprinkle with the crystallised sugar.

	Cal.	Pro.	Fat	Carbo.
Per Serving	180	6.1	5.2	26.6

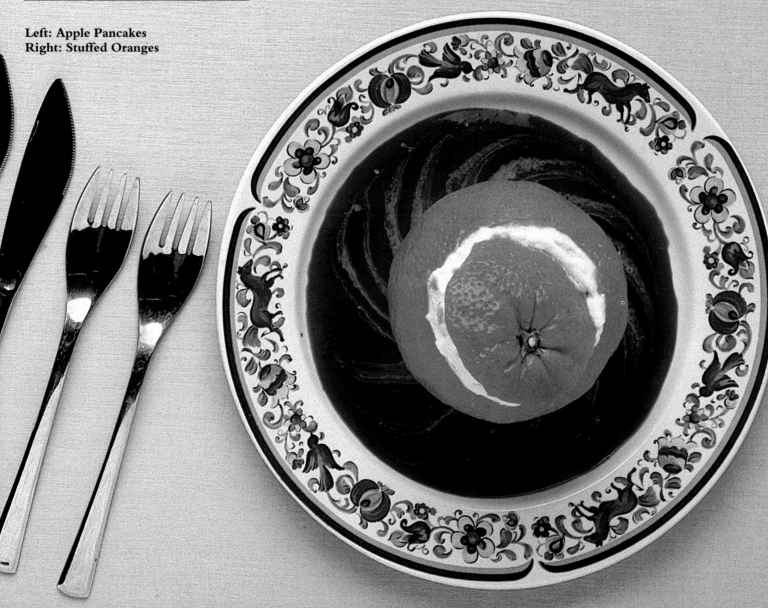

GRAPEFRUIT ICED DRINK

Serves 4

4 grapefruits, squeezed
1 lemon, rind and flesh
4 tablespoons (100g) sugar
¼ litre water
2 egg whites

Put the water, 3 tablespoons of sugar and the lemon rind (without the flesh) in a saucepan and simmer for 10 minutes. Cool. Take out the lemon rind and mix sugar water with the grapefruit juice and flesh of the lemon. Put into the freezer. When half frozen, beat the mixture well and mix it with the egg whites which have been beaten into stiff peaks with the remaining sugar. Return to the freezer, beating again just before serving.

	Cal.	Pro.	Fat	Carbo.
Per Serving	*155*	*2.5*	*0.2*	*36*

Top: Tropical Fruit Salad
Bottom: Chunky Fruit Salad

TROPICAL FRUIT SALAD

Serves 4

200g pineapple
200g raspberries (or strawberries)
200g kiwi fruit
100g banana
2 tablespoons sugar
½ lemon

Divide the pineapple rings into eight pieces. Leave the raspberries whole (or chop the strawberries in half). Cut the kiwi into large pieces. Finely slice the banana; sprinkle the fruit with the sugar and lemon juice, and leave for an hour before serving. Serve cool but not very chilled.

	Cal.	Pro.	Fat	Carbo.
Per Serving	*125*	*1.1*	*0.5*	*29*

CHUNKY FRUIT SALAD

Serves 4

3 oranges
3 apples
3 pears
3 tablespoons sugar
1 lemon

Peel the oranges carefully, removing only the outer skin and not the white pith. Chop the peel into very fine strips, put in cold water and cook for 10 minutes, then drain and change the water (to take away the bitterness). Return to the heat with ¼ litre of water and the 3 tablespoons of sugar. Cook for another 10 minutes and let the syrup cool. Now peel the oranges again, removing all pith and separate into segments.

Peel the apples and cut into large slices to match the size of the orange segments and sprinkle them with lemon juice. Do the same with the pears. Mix all the fruit with the syrup and the strips of orange peel and allow to rest for half an hour before serving. It should be served cool but not chilled to maximise the taste of the fruit.

	Cal.	Pro.	Fat	Carbo.
Per Serving	*153*	*1.2*	*0.7*	*35*

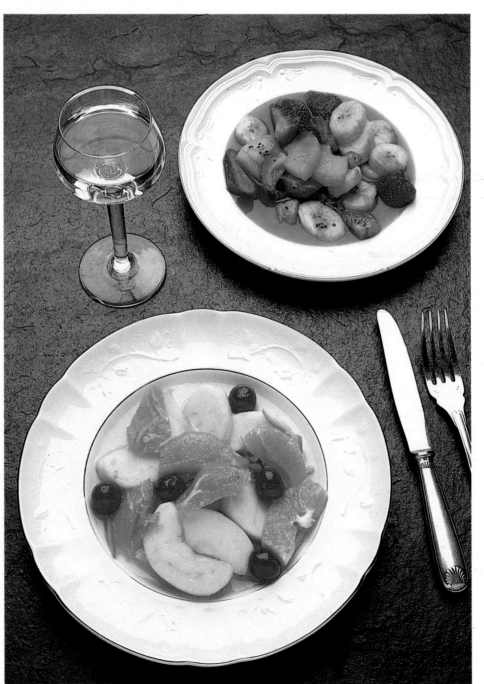